The Integration of Pharmacological and Nonpharmacological Treatments in Drug/Alcohol Addictions

The Integration of Pharmacological and Nonpharmacological Treatments in Drug/Alcohol Addictions has been co-published simultaneously as *Journal of Addictive Diseases*, Volume 16, Number 4 1997.

The *Journal of Addictive Diseases* Monographs/"Separates"
(formerly *Advances in Alcohol & Substance Abuse* series)*

Opiate Receptors, Neurotransmitters, and Drug Dependence: Basic Science-Clinical Correlates, edited by Barry Stimmel*

Recent Advances in the Biology of Alcoholism, edited by Charles S. Lieber and Barry Stimmel*

Effects of Maternal Alcohol and Drug Abuse on the Newborn, edited by Barry Stimmel*

Evaluation of Drug Treatment Programs, edited by Barry Stimmel*

Current Controversies in Alcoholism, edited by Barry Stimmel*

Federal Priorities in Funding Alcohol and Drug Abuse Programs, edited by Barry Stimmel*

Psychosocial Constructs of Alcoholism and Substance Abuse, edited by Barry Stimmel*

The Addictive Behaviors, edited by Howard Shaffer and Barry Stimmel*

Conceptual Issues in Alcoholism and Substance Abuse, edited by Joyce H. Lowinson and Barry Stimmel*

Dual Addiction: Pharmacological Issues in the Treatment of Concomitant Alcoholism and Drug Abuse, edited by Mary Jeanne Kreek and Barry Stimmel*

Cultural and Sociological Aspects of Alcoholism and Substance Abuse, edited by Barry Stimmel*

Alcohol and Drug Abuse in the Affluent, edited by Barry Stimmel*

Alcohol and Substance Abuse in Adolescence, edited by Judith S. Brook, Dan Lettieri, David W. Brook, and Barry Stimmel*

Controversies in Alcoholism and Substance Abuse, edited by Barry Stimmel*

Alcohol and Substance Abuse in Women and Children, edited by Barry Stimmel*

Cocaine: Pharmacology, Addiction, and Therapy, edited by Mark S. Gold, Marc Galanter, and Barry Stimmel*

Children of Alcoholics, edited by Margaret Bean-Bayog and Barry Stimmel*

Pharmacological Issues in Alcohol and Substance Abuse, edited by Barry Stimmel*

AIDS and Substance Abuse, edited by Larry Siegel*

Alcohol Research from Bench to Bedside, edited by Enoch Gordis, Boris Tabakoff, and Markku Linnoila*

Addiction Potential of Abused Drugs and Drug Classes, edited by Carlton K. Erikson, Martin A. Javors, and William W. Morgan*

Behavioral and Biochemical Issues in Substance Abuse, edited by Frank R. George and Doris Clouet*

Cocaine, AIDS, and Intravenous Drug Use, edited by Samuel R. Friedman and Douglas S. Lipton

What Works in Drug Abuse Epidemiology, edited by Blanche Frank and Ronald Simeone

Cocaine: Physiological and Physiopathological Effects, edited by Alfonso Paredes and David A. Gorlick

Comorbidity of Addictive and Psychiatric Disorders, edited by Norman S. Miller

Experimental Therapeutics in Addiction Medicine, edited by Stephen Magura and Andrew Rosenblum

The Effectiveness of Social Interventions for Homeless Substance Abusers, edited by Gerald J. Stahler and Barry Stimmel

The Neurobiology of Cocaine Addiction: From Bench to Bedside, edited by Herman Joseph and Barry Stimmel

Intensive Outpatient Treatment for the Addictions, edited by Edward Gottheil

The Integration of Pharmacological and Nonpharmacological Treatments in Drug/Alcohol Addictions, edited by Norman S. Miller

These books were published simultaneously as special thematic issues of the *Journal of Addictive Diseases* and are available bound separately. Visit Haworth's website at http://www.haworth.com to search our online catalog for complete tables of contents and ordering information for these and other publications. Or call 1-800-HAWORTH (outside US/Canada: 607-722-5857), Fax 1-800-895-0582 (outside US/Canada: 607-771-0012) or e-mail getinfo@haworth.com

The Integration of Pharmacological and Nonpharmacological Treatments in Drug/Alcohol Addictions

Norman S. Miller, MD
Editor

Barry Stimmel, MD
Series Editor

The Integration of Pharmacological and Nonpharmacological Treatments in Drug/Alcohol Addictions has been co-published simultaneously as *Journal of Addictive Diseases*, Volume 16, Number 4 1997.

HMP

The Haworth Medical Press
An Imprint of
The Haworth Press, Inc.
New York • London

Published by

The Haworth Medical Press, 10 Alice Street, Binghamton, NY 13904-1580 USA

The Haworth Medical Press is an imprint of The Haworth Press, Inc., 10 Alice Street, Binghamton, NY 13904-1580 USA.

The Integration of Pharmacological and Nonpharmacological Treatments in Drug/Alcohol Addictions has been co-published simultaneously as *Journal of Addictive Diseases*, Volume 16, Number 4 1997.

Cover design by Thomas J. Mayshock Jr.

Library of Congress Cataloging-in-Publication Data

The integration of pharmacological and nonpharmacological treatments in drug/alcohol addictions / Norman S. Miller, editor.
p. cm.–(Journal of addictive diseases ; v. 16, no. 4)
Has also been published as Journal of addictive diseases, v. 16, no. 4, 1997
Includes bibliographical references and index.
ISBN 0-7890-0375-9 (alk. paper)
1. Substance abuse–Treatment. 2. Substance abuse–Chemotherapy. I. Miller, Norman S. II. Journal of addictive diseases. III. Series.
[DNLM: 1. Substance Dependence–therapy. 2. Alcoholism–therapy. 3. Psychopharmacology. W1 JO533PU v. 16 no. 4 1997 / WM 270 I593 1997]
RC564.I55 1997
616.86'06–dc21 97-31682
CIP

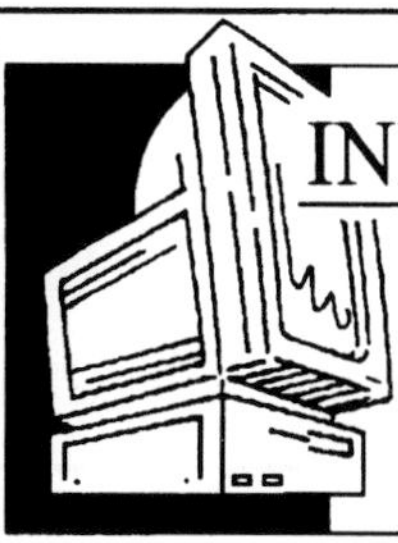

INDEXING & ABSTRACTING

Contributions to this publication are selectively indexed or abstracted in print, electronic, online, or CD-ROM version(s) of the reference tools and information services listed below. This list is current as of the copyright date of this publication. See the end of this section for additional notes.

- ***Abstracts in Anthropology,*** Baywood Publishing Company, 26 Austin Avenue, P.O. Box 337, Amityville, NY 11701
- ***Abstracts of Research in Pastoral Care & Counseling,*** Loyola College, 7135 Minstrel Way, Suite 101, Columbia, MD 21045
- ***Academic Abstracts/CD-ROM,*** EBSCO Publishing Editorial Department, P.O. Box 590, Ipswich, MA 01938-0590
- ***ADDICTION ABSTRACTS,*** National Addiction Centre, 4 Windsor Walk, London SE5 8AF, England
- ***ALCONLINE Database,*** Centralforbundet for Alcohol-och narkotikaupplysning, Box 70412, Stockholm, Sweden
- ***Behavioral Medicine Abstracts,*** University of Washington, Department of Social Work & Speech & Hearing Sciences, Box 354900, Seattle, WA 98195
- ***Biosciences Information Service of Biological Abstracts (BIOSIS),*** Biosciences Information Service, 2100 Arch Street, Philadelphia, PA 19103-1399
- ***Brown University Digest of Addiction Theory and Application, The (DATA Newsletter),*** Project Cork Institute, Dartmouth Medical School, 14 South Main Street, Suite 2F, Hanover, NH 03755-2015
- ***Cambridge Scientific Abstracts,*** Health & Safety Science Abstracts, 7200 Wisconsin Avenue #601, Bethesda, MD 20814
- ***Child Development Abstracts & Bibliography,*** University of Kansas, 2 Bailey Hall, Lawrence, KS 66045
- ***CNPIEC Reference Guide: Chinese National Directory of Foreign Periodicals,*** P.O. Box 88, Beijing, Peoples Republic of China
- ***Criminal Justice Abstracts,*** Willow Tree Press, 15 Washington Street, 4th Floor, Newark, NJ 07102
- ***Criminal Justice Periodical Index,*** University Microfilms, Inc., P.O. Box 32770, Louisville, KY 40232

(continued)

- ***Criminology, Penology and Police Science Abstracts,*** Kugler Publications, P.O. Box 11188, 1001 GD Amsterdam, The Netherlands
- ***Current Contents . . . .*** see: ***Institute for Scientific Information***
- ***Educational Administration Abstracts (EAA),*** Sage Publications, Inc., 2455 Teller Road, Newbury Park, CA 91320
- ***Excerpta Medica/Secondary Publishing Division,*** Elsevier Science Inc., Secondary Publishing Division, 655 Avenue of the Americas, New York, NY 10010
- ***Family Studies Database (online and CD/ROM),*** National Information Services Corporation, 306 East Baltimore Pike, 2nd Floor, Media, PA 19063
- ***Health Source: Indexing & Abstracting of 160 selected health related journals, updated monthly,*** EBSCO Publishing, 83 Pine Street, Peabody, MA 01960
- ***Health Source Plus: expanded version of "Health Source" to be released shortly:*** EBSCO Publishing, 83 Pine Street, Peabody, MA 01960
- ***Index Medicus,*** National Library of Medicine, 8600 Rockville Pike, Bethesda, MD 20894
- ***Index to Periodical Articles Related to Law,*** University of Texas, 727 East 26th Street, Austin, TX 78705
- ***Institute for Scientific Information,*** 3501 Market Street, Philadelphia, Pennsylvania 19104. Coverage in:
  a) Social Science Citation Index (SSCI): print, online, CD-ROM
  b) Research Alerts (current awareness service)
  c) Social SciSearch (magnetic tape)
  d) Current Contents/Social & Behavioral Sciences (weekly current awareness service)
- ***International Pharmaceutical Abstracts,*** ASHP, 7272 Wisconsin Avenue, Bethesda, MD 20814
- ***INTERNET ACCESS (& additional networks) Bulletin Board for Libraries ("BUBL"), coverage of information resources on INTERNET, JANET, and other networks.***
  - <URL:http://bubl.ac.uk/>
  - The new locations will be found under <URL:http://bubl.ac.uk/link/>.
  - Any existing BUBL users who have problems finding information on the new service should contact the BUBL help line by sending e-mail to <bubl@bubl.ac.uk>.

  The Andersonian Library, Curran Building, 101 St. James Road, Glasgow G4 0NS, Scotland
- ***Medication Use STudies (MUST) Database,*** The University of Mississippi, School of Pharmacy, University, MS 38677

(continued)

- ***Mental Health Abstracts (online through DIALOG),*** IFI/Plenum Data Company, 3202 Kirkwood Highway, Wilmington, DE 19808
- ***NIAAA Alcohol and Alcohol Problems Science Database (ETOH),*** National Institute on Alcohol Abuse and Alcoholism, 1400 Eye Street NW, Suite 600, Washington, DC 20005
- ***PASCAL, c/o Institute de L'Information Scientifique et Technique,*** Cross-disciplinary electronic database covering the fields of science, technology & medicine. Also available on CD-ROM, and can generate customized retrospective searches. For more information: INIST, Customer Desk, 2, allee du Parc de Brabois, F-54514 Vandoeuvre Cedex, France, http//wwwinist.fr
- ***Psychological Abstracts (PsycINFO),*** American Psychological Association, P.O. Box 91600, Washington, DC 20090-1600
- ***Sage Family Studies Abstracts (SFSA),*** Sage Publications, Inc., 2455 Teller Road, Newbury Park, CA 91320
- ***Sage Urban Studies Abstracts (SUSA),*** Sage Publications, Inc., 2455 Teller Road, Newbury Park, CA 91320
- ***Social Planning/Policy & Development Abstracts (SOPODA),*** Sociological Abstracts, Inc., P.O. Box 22206, San Diego, CA 92192-0206
- ***Social Work Abstracts,*** National Association of Social Workers, 750 First Street NW, 8th Floor, Washington, DC 20002
- ***Sociological Abstracts (SA),*** Sociological Abstracts, Inc., P.O. Box 22206, San Diego, CA 92192-0206
- ***SOMED (social medicine) Database,*** Landes Institut fur Den Offentlichen Gesundheitsdienst NRW, Postfach 20 10 12, D-33548 Bielefeld, Germany
- ***Studies on Women Abstracts,*** Carfax Publishing Company, P.O. Box 25, Abingdon, Oxon, OX14 3UE, United Kingdom
- ***Violence and Abuse Abstracts: A Review of Current Literature on Interpersonal Violence (VAA),*** Sage Publications, Inc., 2455 Teller Road, Newbury Park, CA 91320

(continued)

SPECIAL BIBLIOGRAPHIC NOTES

related to special journal issues (separates) and indexing/abstracting

- ❑ indexing/abstracting services in this list will also cover material in any "separate" that is co-published simultaneously with Haworth's special thematic journal issue or DocuSerial. Indexing/abstracting usually covers material at the article/chapter level.
- ❑ monographic co-editions are intended for either non-subscribers or libraries which intend to purchase a second copy for their circulating collections.
- ❑ monographic co-editions are reported to all jobbers/wholesalers/approval plans. The source journal is listed as the "series" to assist the prevention of duplicate purchasing in the same manner utilized for books-in-series.
- ❑ to facilitate user/access services all indexing/abstracting services are encouraged to utilize the co-indexing entry note indicated at the bottom of the first page of each article/chapter/contribution.
- ❑ this is intended to assist a library user of any reference tool (whether print, electronic, online, or CD-ROM) to locate the monographic version if the library has purchased this version but not a subscription to the source journal.
- ❑ individual articles/chapters in any Haworth publication are also available through the Haworth Document Delivery Service (HDDS).

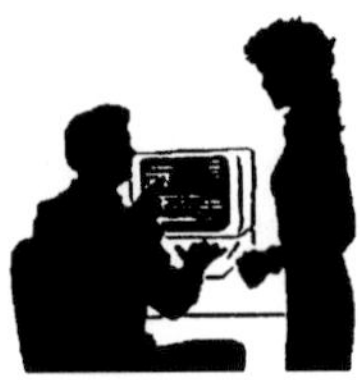

The Integration of Pharmacological and Nonpharmacological Treatments in Drug/Alcohol Addictions

CONTENTS

∞ ALL HAWORTH MEDICAL PRESS BOOKS AND JOURNALS ARE PRINTED ON CERTIFIED ACID-FREE PAPER

ABOUT THE EDITOR

Norman S. Miller, PhD, is Chief of Division of Addictions Programs, Associate Professor of Psychiatry and Neurology in the College of Medicine, and Research Psychiatrist in the Psychiatric Institute for Research at The University of Illinois at Chicago. Dr. Miller has filled many professional positions, including Regional Director of the Midwest Region and Chair of the Dual Diagnosis and Nomenclature Committees for the American Society for Addiction Medicine (ASAM) and Regional Director for the Ruth Fox Endowment. He is a fellow in the American Psychopathological Association and a member of the American Psychiatric Association, the American Society for Addiction Medicine, and the American Academy of Psychiatrists in Alcoholism and Addictions. He is also currently a member of the Task Force on Treatment for the Office of National Drug Control Policy (ONDCI), Office of the President of the United States; a member of the Center for Substance Abuse Treatment (CSAT) on Screening, Assessment, and Treatment Planning for Patients with Coexisting Mental Illness and Alcohol and Other Drug (AOD) Abuse: and co-chair of the Task Force for Undergraduate Medical Education, AMERSA (Association for Medical Education and Research in Substance Abuse). Dr. Miller is Medical Advisor for the Department of Alcohol and Substance Abuse. State of Illinois, and a public member of the Illinois Marriage and Family Therapy Examining and Disciplinary Board for the Department of Professional Regulation and the Governor Jim Edgar Administration. Editor of *Principles of Addiction Medicine* (First Edition) and author of 220 medical/scientific articles, book chapters, and reviews, and 11 books on Addiction Medicine, he appears in *Who's Who in America* and *Who's Who International.*

EDITORIAL

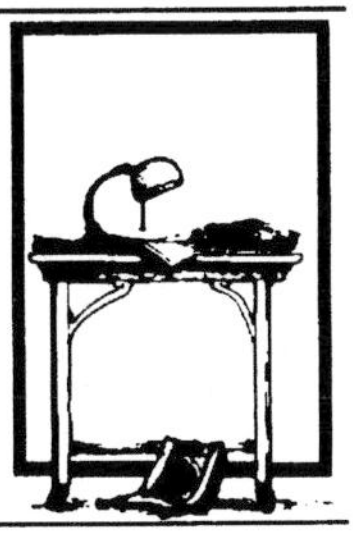

The Integration of Pharmacological and Nonpharmacological Treatments in Drug/Alcohol Addiction

The "integration of pharmacological and nonpharmacological treatments" is not new to Addiction Medicine. The use of medications for detoxification is well integrated in the standard of care for withdrawal from drugs that produce pharmacological dependence. Medications for the treatment of drug withdrawal reduce morbidity and mortality and improve engagement and compliance with psychosocial therapies. Generally detoxification with medications has

[Haworth co-indexing entry note]: "The Integration of Pharmacological and Nonpharmacological Treatments in Drug/Alcohol Addiction." Miller, Norman S. Co-published simultaneously in *Journal of Addictive Diseases* (The Haworth Medical Press, an imprint of The Haworth Press, Inc.) Vol. 16, No. 4, 1997, pp. 1-5; and: *The Integration of Pharmacological and Nonpharmacological Treatments in Drug/Alcohol Addictions* (ed: Norman S. Miller, and Barry Stimmel) The Haworth Medical Press, an imprint of The Haworth Press, Inc., 1997, pp. 1-5. Single or multiple copies of this article are available for a fee from The Haworth Document Delivery Service [1-800-342-9678, 9:00 a.m. - 5:00 p.m. (EST). E-mail address: getinfo@haworth.com].

been intended for the acute phase lasting hours to days following cessation of drug use.[1,2]

Our recent efforts in the development of medications have extended the treatment time frame to months following drug use. This is aimed at the prevention of relapse. However, the search for such medications is not new as clinicians and researchers have long tried numerous agents aimed at decreasing and eliminating drug use. Our efforts to date have taught us some humbling lessons about addictive diseases, namely, that they are complex biopsychosocial entities which defy simple "either/or" solutions. Rigid dogma will not answer these questions nor improve treatment for our patients. Moreover, clearly conceived rationales derived from principles and practices in Addiction Medicine will be required if research efforts are to be relevant to patient care. We need a step by step progression from research findings to the development of clinical standards to produce effective medications.[2-5] Unfortunately, much research to date often has not incorporated basic medical concepts that are important to evaluate outcome in response to medication trials. More sensitive and specific criteria for defining outcome from addictive diseases is needed.

The continued use of the term *abuse* does little to foster medication development and should be discontinued. Addiction consists of: (1) preoccupation with acquiring alcohol/drugs (drug seeking), (2) compulsive use (continued use despite adverse consequences), and (3) a pattern of relapse after abstinence is achieved. Loss of control over the use of alcohol and drugs is central to the definition of addiction and pervasive to its behaviors. Recently, the basis of the behavioral definition of addiction has been located in neurobiological drive states in the substrate of the limbic system (mesolimbic pathway projections of dopamine neurons to the nucleus accumbens in the limbic forebrain).[6] The physiology of withdrawal has also been clearly defined in norepinephrine pathways in the locus ceruleus that projects from the pons diffusely to central and peripheral sites.

We have effective psychosocial treatment for addictive disease. We can obtain one year abstinence rates of 60% following abstinence-based forms of treatment. Moreover, these abstinence rates can be increased with compliance with continuing care or 12-step attendance. While these compliance rates compare favorably to other medical treatments, e.g., hypertension (30%), we can hope to improve these figures by integrating medications with psychosocial treatments subsequent to detoxification. The assumption is that increased compliance will lead to increased abstinence.[7,8,9]

The articles in this issue attempt to summarize and provide groundwork for future considerations in developing and integrating medications with the standard of care for addictions treatment. The neurobiological targets known to date are reviewed toward the view that rationale development will proceed according to substrates that subserve all addictive behaviors, recognizing that addiction to one addicting drug will increase the likelihood of addiction to others.[10] The treatment with medications used for comorbid psychiatric disorders is also increasingly important as high rates of addictive use of alcohol and drugs are found in many psychiatric disorders, particularly, those that require psychotropic medications, e.g., schizophrenic and bipolar disorders. Medications aimed at dopamine pathways could possibly treat both categories as the mesolimbic pathway has been implicated in schizophrenic as well as addictive disorders.[11] This overlap in neurochemical pathways suggests a common vulnerability as well.[12]

We will need sharper definitions of abstinence and recovery that include active participation by the individual.[13] We live in a smaller world and Addiction Medicine is no exception. We have included a summary of the European experience in medication development, particularly acamprosate, which has shown promise in reducing alcohol use in multisite trials. In many ways Europe is following the United States in developing psychosocial treatments for addictive disorders and their success in the U.S. has been recognized.[14] The issue ends with queries about our direction in medication development, with its promises and pitfalls.[15]

The core integration of medicines with recovery will require a careful rethinking of basic tenets for both pharmacological and nonpharmacological approaches. The "clean and sober" approach will have to be re-examined and perhaps modified to add a "drug" solution. Similarly, the obsession of the addict that a drug solution will solve their addictive drug use will have to be tempered to include those drugs that are therapeutic without significant addiction potential. We also will have to shift from an all or nothing position in evaluating medications to one where we weigh risks and benefits of specific therapies. Most areas of medicine tolerate a balance between "good and bad"; however, knowledge and skill are required for an adequate evaluation. An evaluator will have to differentiate compliance in therapeutic use from addictive drug use. This is not easy as to date the literature on benzodiazepines suggests that most researchers and clinicians still cannot tell the difference between addiction, tolerance and dependence to benzodiazepines as very few assess addictive use.

The use of medications for prevention of relapse in addictive illness challenges some firmly held beliefs regarding abstinence as a foundation for recovery, or its necessity to have enduring and maturational changes preventing relapse. As an example, recent studies on naltrexone defined relapse as 5 or more drinks of alcohol for men and 4 or more for women. Continuous abstinence was not a consistently significant finding for the effects of naltrexone. Additional research is needed to determine if short-term benefits of reduced drinking will parlay to long-term reduction in morbidity and mortality, which we know from studies result from abstinence to alcohol and other drugs.

Of course, such integration can be enhanced by research. We have learned from our experience in Addiction Medicine that whatever is derived from research must conform to the standard of care and be able to be integrated into medical practice. Ignoring these realities will leave researchers pondering why clinicians will not incorporate new findings into clinical practice. Clinicians in Addiction Medicine are looking toward researchers to help solve clinical problems and to develop new strategies to improve clinical care. Failure to integrate research with practice and pharmacologic with nonpharmacologic therapies will ill serve all in the field especially our patients who deserve our best efforts to reduce morbidity and mortality from addictive disease.

Norman S. Miller, MD

REFERENCES

1. Miller NS, ed. Principles of addiction medicine. Washington, D.C.: American Society of Addiction Medicine, 1994.

2. Litten RZ, Allen JP. Pharmacotherapies for alcoholism: promising agents and clinical issues. Alcohol Clin Exp Res. 1991; 15(4):620-33.

3. Volpicelli J, Atterman A, Hayashida M, et al. Naltrexone in the treatment of alcohol dependence. Arch Gen Psychiatry. 1992; 49:876-80.

4. Mason B, Ritro E, Morgan R, et al. A double-blind placebo-controlled pilot study to evaluate the efficacy and safety of oral nalmetene HCl for alcohol dependence. Alcohol Clin Exp Res. 1994; 18:1162-7.

5. Consensus Conference on the Neuropharmacology of Alcohol Dependence and the Role of Pharmacotherapy in its Treatment. Alcohol Alcohol. 1996; 31(Suppl 1):1-87.

6. Jaffe JH. Drug and addiction abuse. In: Gilman AG, Goodman LS, Rall TW, Murad F, eds. The pharmacological basis of therapeutics, 7th ed. New York: Macmillan, 1985:532-81.

7. Miller NS, ed. Treatment of the addictions. Applications of outcome research for clinical management. New York: Haworth Press, 1995.

8. Miller NS, Gold MS, Smith DE, eds. Manual of therapeutics for addictions. New York: John Wiley & Sons, Inc., 1997.

9. Walsh EC, Hingson RW, Merrigan DM, et al. A randomized trial of treatment options for alcohol abusing workers. N Engl J Med. 1991; 325:775-82.

10. Miller NS, Guttman JC, Chawla S. Integration of generalized vulnerability to drug and alcohol addiction. J Addict Dis. 1997; 16(4):7-22.

11. Pechter BM, Miller NS. Psychopharmacotherapy for addictive and comorbid disorders: current studies. J Addict Dis. 1997; 16(4):23-40.

12. Huber A, Ling W, Shoptaw S, Gulati V, Brethen P, Rawson R. Integrating treatments for methamphetamine abuse: a psychosocial perspective. J Addict Dis. 1997; 16(4):41-50.

13. Miller NS, Smith DE. The integration of pharmacotherapy and nonpharmacotherapy. J Addict Dis. 1997; 16(4):51-64.

14. Poldrugo F. Integration of pharmacotherapies in the existing programs for the treatment of alcoholics: an international perspective. J Addict Dis. 1997; 16(4):65-82.

15. Ling W, Shoptaw S. Integration of research in pharmacotherapy for addictive disease: Where are we? Where are we going? J Addict Dis. 1997; 16(4):83-102.

Integration of Generalized Vulnerability to Drug and Alcohol Addiction

Norman S. Miller, MD
Jane C. Guttman, BA
Soyna Chawla, MD

SUMMARY. The vulnerability to develop addiction to alcohol has been well established in familial and genetic studies. Similar familial and genetic studies have supported a vulnerability to drug addiction. The co-occurrence of alcohol and drug addiction in the same individuals is highly prevalent in clinical populations. Common putative neurochemical mechanisms underlie addiction to both alcohol and drugs, namely, in the mesolimbic pathway and the locus ceruleus in the brain. Treatment strategies are directed at both alcohol and multiple drug addictions in patient populations. The formulation of a generalized vulnerability that extends to both alcohol and drug addiction is not only possible but necessary to explain the substantial numbers of individuals who develop both alcohol and drug addictions. Future research that is pertinent and relevant may depend on the understanding of a generalized vulnerability to develop alcohol and drug addiction and its application in diagnostic strategies and treatment models. *[Article copies available for a fee from The Haworth Document Delivery Service: 1-800-342-9678. E-mail address: getinfo@haworth.com]*

Norman S. Miller, Jane C. Guttman, and Soyna Chawla are affiliated with the Department of Psychiatry, The University of Illinois at Chicago, Chicago, IL.

Address correspondence to: Norman S. Miller, MD, The University of Illinois at Chicago, Department of Psychiatry (M/C 913), 912 South Wood Street, Chicago, IL 60612-7327.

[Haworth co-indexing entry note]: "Integration of Generalized Vulnerability to Drug and Alcohol Addiction." Miller, Norman S., Jane C. Guttman, and Soyna Chawla. Co-published simultaneously in *Journal of Addictive Diseases* (The Haworth Medical Press, an imprint of The Haworth Press, Inc.) Vol. 16, No. 4, 1997, pp. 7-22; and: *The Integration of Pharmacological and Nonpharmacological Treatments in Drug/Alcohol Addictions* (ed: Norman S. Miller, and Barry Stimmel) The Haworth Medical Press, an imprint of The Haworth Press, Inc., 1997, pp. 7-22. Single or multiple copies of this article are available for a fee from The Haworth Document Delivery Service [1-800-342-9678, 9:00 a.m. - 5:00 p.m. (EST). E-mail address: getinfo@haworth.com].

COMMON BIOLOGICAL INTERACTIONS IN ADDICTIVE DRUG/ALCOHOL USE

Several neurotransmitters may be involved in the various appetitive systems that underlie addictive behaviors. In studies, the major neurotransmitters identified in drug and alcohol addiction are the opioid peptides, dopamine, serotonin, and norepinephrine. These neurotransmitters have individual and interactive relationships in the reinforcement center and with the instinctual drive states in the brain. Together, this center and the drive states are thought to generate and underlie addictive use of drugs and alcohol.[1] Recent findings have suggested that the common denominator for a wide range of classes of addictive drugs is their ability to activate the dopaminergic fibers in the mesolimbic system.[2,3]

The reinforcement center has been shown to contain dopamine neurons that project from their location in the ventral tegmentum to the mesolimbic system in the forebrain. Opiate receptors were found on these dopamine neurons and stimulation with opiates activated this dopamine system. Self-administration studies have shown that stimulation of the mesolimbic area supports addictive use of heroin, cocaine, nicotine, and ethanol. Blockade of dopamine receptors prevented the self-administration of opiates and cocaine, and blockade of norepinephrine sites reduces alcohol intake. Also, antagonism with narcotic blocking agents attenuated reinforcement behavior from cocaine, heroin, and ethanol administration.[3,4] The nature of biological traits and capacity for reward systems in the pathophysiology of nicotine dependence is not wholly clear but studies indicate that nicotine acts on the dopamine neurons in the ventral tegmentum in a fashion similar to other addicting drugs.[5,6]

Other neurotransmitters may be involved in drug and alcohol use and addiction by serving a modulatory function. In humans, administration of serotonin (5HT) reuptake inhibitors (zimelidine, fluoxetine, citlopram) to nondepressed heavy-alcohol-consumers and alcoholics was associated with a reduction in the number of drinks consumed and increase in abstinent days.[7] A possible rationale is the influence of serotonin on other neurotransmitter systems. Serotonin neurons in the hypothalamus project to the metencephalon neurons that inhibit mesencephalic endogenous opiate peptides and projections of gamma-aminobutyric acid (GABA) neurons. It has been demonstrated that GABA neurons interact to inhibit dopamine neurons in the ventral tegmentum and other neurotransmitters and in doing so also perform widespread modulation functions.[8]

Lab studies suggest a variability in development of selectivity and tolerance of nicotine and on sensitivity to nicotine, suggesting a genetic basis on rewarding effects of nicotine. Newer studies indicate that cigarette smoking has a heritability index of 53%. Nicotine dependence may also be related to high initial sensitivity to nicotine leading to an increased tolerance in susceptible individuals.[5,6] (See Figure 1.)

THEORETICAL IMPLICATIONS

The theoretical implications extend to concepts of generalized biological vulnerability for drug and alcohol addiction. The co-oc-

FIGURE 1. Schematic drawing of the possible interactions between the endogenous opioid system and the brain nuclei responsible for the mediation of the positive reinforcing effects of ethanol. *Adapted from* Gianoulakis C. Implication of endogenous opioids and dopamine in alcoholism: human and basic science studies. Alcohol Alcohol. 1996; 31 (Suppl. 1):33:-42.

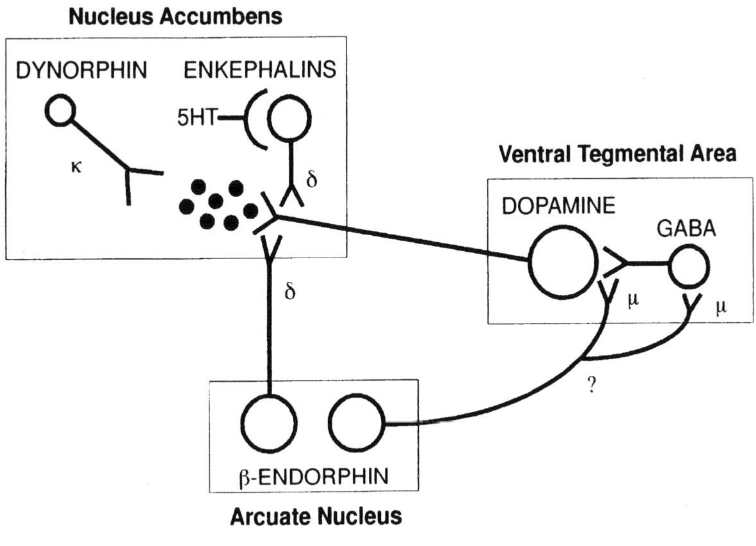

currence of multiple drug and alcohol addictions and their common transmission in the adoption, twin, and familial studies suggest a genetic predisposition inclusive of a wide range of drugs and alcohol.[9-11] While studies are inconclusive at this point, they do indicate the genetic transmission for drugs may be similar to that for alcohol. Moreover, the genetic influence appears to be operative for both alcohol and drug addiction in the same individual and groups of ostensibly dissimilar individuals. These findings are consistent with the clinical observations that alcohol and drugs can be used interchangeably in the addictive mode and that distinct hierarchical combinations are apparent, although alcohol is pervasive throughout subtypes.[12-16] It is important to examine current and future generations of alcoholics and drug addicts for transmission of specific or common drug types (alcohol) in adoption, twin, and family cases. It is important to continue to assess for the combined alcohol and drug use/dependence in the multiply addicted for epidemiology, diagnosis, and treatment implications. It is also important to continue to elucidate common brain mechanisms that underlie generalized biological vulnerabilities and identify specific brain targets for subtypes of alcohol and drug addiction for future treatments.

More research studies distinguishing between genetic and environmental determinants are necessary. Investigations of genetic and familial patterns of generational transmission of drugs and alcohol in relation to environmental influences regarding exposure to alcohol and drugs are needed. In a simplified formula, the addiction rate can be equated to vulnerability plus exposure: genetic factors pertain to vulnerability whereas environmental factors relate to exposure. For the immediate future, prevention and treatment may be more easily accomplished by manipulation of the environment than by genetic alteration, whereas knowledge of genetic factors will provide direction for therapeutic agents for addictive disorders and genetic counseling.[17]

TREATMENT IMPLICATIONS

The studies to date strongly suggest that treatment of drug and alcohol addiction must be aimed at both drugs and alcohol, in part because of apparent genetically determined common biological mechanisms. The treatment of only a single drug addiction reduces the probability of achieving a successful outcome. Generally, it is advisable that drug addicts and alcoholics abstain from all drugs due to the potential for developing further addictions. Although not well documented, clinical experience confirms that cocaine addicts frequently relapse to cocaine because of the use of alcohol or cannabis before using cocaine. Also, opiate addicts often relapse to alcohol or other drugs with or without returning to addictive use of opiates. Alcoholics may resort to using other drugs such as benzodiazepines addictively before eventually relapsing to alcohol.

Both pharmacologic and nonpharmacologic treatments for drug and alcohol addiction will benefit from a full appreciation and understanding of multiple drug and alcohol dependence and biological vulnerabilities.[18] Medications targeted for only drug or alcohol addiction will have limited efficacy, as will the abstinence-based 12-step programs, behavioral, social, and cognitive therapies, if only alcohol or single drug types are the object of treatment.[19,20]

PREVALENCE OF DEPENDENCE IN TREATMENT POPULATIONS

In treatment populations of adults and adolescents, between 70 to 90% of cocaine addicts, 50 to 70% of opiate (heroin and methadone) addicts, 20 to 50% of benzodiazepine addicts, and 80 to 90% of cannabis addicts were alcoholics. Moreover, in other studies, 20 to 50% of opiate addicts were cocaine, benzodiazepine, and cannabis addicts.[20]

Many studies of alcoholics and drug addicts in treatment populations have found that in both groups, alcohol is often the first drug used addictively. Moreover, more than two drug diagnoses were present in the majority of those addicted to alcohol, in addition to, in decreasing frequency, nicotine, cannabis, cocaine, benzodiazepines, hallucinogens, and opiates. In adolescents and young adults, a triad of alcohol, marijuana, and cocaine addiction was a common occurrence.[21-23] The natural history of alcohol dependence is highly variable and age dependent as the young alcoholic begins using alcohol in early teenage years (ages 13 to 15) and progresses to addictive use of alcohol by the age of 15 or 16. A year or two after the onset of alcohol addiction, other drugs such as nicotine, cannabis, cocaine, opiates, and hallucinogens are used addictively. The addictive use of sedative/hypnotic drugs does not appear to show an age effect as they are used equally at all ages but greater among women than among men by perhaps a ratio of 2:3.[24]

GENETIC STUDIES

Adoption Studies: Alcoholism

Several adoption studies showed that sons of alcoholics raised by adoptive parents became alcoholics significantly more often than sons of nonalcoholics raised by adoptive parents. Similar results of three separate adoption studies conducted in Denmark, Sweden, and the United States (Iowa), and a half-sibling study revealed the following:

1. Sons of alcoholics were 3 to 4 times more likely to become alcoholics than were sons of nonalcoholics, whether the sons of alcoholics were raised by their alcoholic biologic parents or by their nonalcoholic adoptive parents. The studies can be criticized on the basis of small numbers of subjects, criteria for diagnosis of alcoholism, and overlap between numbers of alcoholic parents of alcoholic and nonalcoholic adoptees. Nonetheless, the composite results and replication in additional studies strongly support an inheritance in the development of alcoholism.[25-27]
2. Sons of alcoholics raised by nonalcoholic adoptive parents were no more susceptible to nonalcoholic adult psychiatric diagnoses than were sons of nonalcoholics raised by nonalcoholic adoptive parents. The Iowa study did find a higher rate of childhood conduct disorder in male offspring of alcoholics.[28]
3. The results regarding female alcoholism were more equivocal. One Danish study[29] found that 4% of the daughters of alcoholics were alcoholics, but 4% of the control women also were alcoholic, introducing the possibility that adoption may contribute to alcoholism. A Swedish study[30] found a low rate of alcoholism in the adopted-out daughters of alcoholics, al-

though a subsequent analysis found a correspondence between alcoholism in the biologic mothers and alcoholism in the adopted-out daughters.[31] The Iowa study also shows a genetic effect in female alcoholism.[28]

4. Alcoholism and antisocial personality were genetically independent disorders for both males and females. The results of the Iowa study showed specificity of inheritance of antisocial and alcoholic conditions, with two types of independent predispositions, one toward alcohol and the other toward antisocial personality.[28]

Adoption: Drug Addiction

An adoption study of genetic and environmental factors in drug abuse revealed that a biological background of alcohol problems predicted increased drug abuse in adoptees. Also, environmental factors, divorce, and psychiatric disturbance in the adoptive family were associated with increased drug abuse.[32]

Twin Studies: Alcoholism

A Finnish study (11,500 twin pairs) and a Swedish study (7,500 male pairs) showed drinking problems were greater in monozygotic twins than in dizygotic twins. Swedish (174 male pairs) and American (15,924 male twins) studies showed that a diagnosis of alcoholism was more concordant in monozygotic twins than in dizygotic twins. Only one study done in England, and which had the smallest number of twin pairs (56 twin pairs) of all the studies, did not show a difference in alcohol behavior between monozygotic twins and dizygotic twins.[25]

A more recent study in a U.S. treatment sample of 50 monozygotic and 64 dizygotic male twins and 31 monozygotic and 24 dizygotic female twins showed a significantly greater concordance rate for alcohol dependence in male and female twins and for alcohol abuse in males only.[33]

Studies of daughters of alcoholics raised by nonalcoholic adoptive parents have been equivocal in regards to supporting heritability of alcoholism in females.[25-27]

Twin Studies: Drug Addiction

In a recent U.S. study, only male monozygotic twins were significantly more concordant than dizygotic twins for other drug abuse/dependence and any substance abuse/dependence including alcohol dependence. However, the ratios of monozygotic to dizygotic concordance were comparable in the two sexes, suggesting that lack of significance in the female sample may be due to low statistical power.[34]

Human twin studies suggest an influence of genetic factors on smoking behaviors including the amount of tobacco smoked. A recent review of 18 twin studies found that the concordance rates for smokers were higher in monozygotic twins than dizygotic twins—even when the twins were raised separately. Evidence suggests that smoking status and magnitude of dependence have independent risk factors.[5,6]

FAMILIAL STUDIES

Familial Alcoholism: Alcoholism

The familial prevalence of alcoholism among male alcoholics has been well documented in large studies. The rate of familial alcoholism is 50% according to most studies, and if an alcoholic reported having one close relative who was alcoholic, he more often than the nonalcoholic reported having two or more relatives with alcoholism.[25,35-38]

Several studies have reported that younger alcoholics have alcoholic relatives more often than older alcoholics, and that familial alcoholics show the first signs of dependence at a younger age than do nonfamilial alcoholics.[25,37] Moreover, familial alcoholics tend to have an earlier age of onset and a more severe form of addiction with a more rapid fulminating course.[25,37] Among 2,215 male alcoholics treated for alcoholism, those with a family history of alcoholism did worse in treatment than did those with no family history; furthermore, the greater number of relatives with alcoholism, the worse the prognosis.[35]

Familial Alcoholism: Drug Addiction

Familial alcoholism among drug addicts is less studied but some data are available. The rate of familial alcoholism was 50% among males and 80% for females in a retrospective study of 150 cocaine dependents. In a prospective study the rate for familial alcoholism was 52% in male and 60% in female cocaine dependents.[39]

Opiate dependents with a parental history of alcoholism were more frequently diagnosed with concurrent alcoholism. In one study 638 opiate dependents with a diagnosis of alcohol dependence had at least one parent with alcohol dependence in 21.3% of the families. Four hundred twenty-two opiate dependents without the diagnosis of alcohol dependence had a 12.5% rate of alcohol dependence in their families. Among the opiate dependents with alcohol dependence, those with parental alcoholism had more severe problems with alcohol.[40]

The results of this study are supportive of both familial and nonfamilial alcoholism in opiate addicts. Because alcoholism is high among opiate addicts at rates of 50 to 75%, an increased rate of familial alcoholism among those opiate addicts with alcoholism may be significant.

Familial Alcohol and Drug Use/Addiction

Two hundred sixty-two adolescents, ages 13 through 17, and one of the parents of each adolescent were interviewed separately in a study on the impact of parental drug and alcohol use on adolescent behavior. The frequency of parental drinking directly correlated with greater drug and alcohol use in the offspring; 72% of the fathers and 77% of the mothers who took one or more drinks of beer or wine per day had offspring who used drugs and alcohol. Those parents who drank beer or wine less than once a month or not at all were much less likely to have adolescent children who used drugs and alcohol. There was a strong relationship found between parental use of marijuana/hashish and adolescent drug and alcohol use. Eighty-one percent of the fathers and 78% of the mothers who used marijuana/hashish had children who used drugs and alcohol.[41]

In a longitudinal study, 82% of drinking families raised youths who also drank, while 72% of abstaining families produced abstainers. Not only did youth behavior approximate parental behavior, but there is a generalization effect as youths used a greater variety of drugs than parents did.[42] Less consistent, however, is the evidence concerning which parent, father or mother, was more influential. A high correlation between a father's alcohol use and the use of alcohol, marijuana, and other drugs by his offspring has been reported. Among African-Americans, a mother's alcohol use is correlated with juvenile drug and alcohol use.[43]

In a sample of 1,380 youths that were examined in the teenage years between the ages of 12 and 18, data regarding the alcohol- and drug-using behaviors were obtained for a positive or negative history of alcoholism for offspring. The offspring with a family history of alcoholism were compared for early differences in patterns of alcohol and drug use with offspring without a family history of alcoholism (having drinking nonalcoholic families, high-stress families, and symptom-free families). No differences were found in several indicators of problem use (early onset of intoxication, frequent intoxication, and escape drinking). However, the analysis did indicate that adolescent alcoholics with a history of familial alcoholism were more likely than family-history-negative adolescents from symptom-free families to report experiencing problems/consequences relating to both drug use and drinking. Significantly, familial alcoholics had rates of self-reported alcohol and/or drug problems about twice that for nonfamilial alcoholics for both males and females.[44,45]

Common vs. Specific Transmission of Drug and Alcohol Use and Dependence in Families

The questions of familial transmission of nonalcohol drug use/dependence in combination and for specific drug types, and with and without alcohol use/dependence, has been not completely studied. Scherer (1971) (76 subjects) showed a high correlation between tranquilizer use in parents and both tranquilizer and cannabis use in offspring.[46] Fawzy, Coombs, and Gerber (1983) (262 subjects) found a 78% prevalence of drug use in adolescent children of parents who admitted using marijuana and hashish.[47] Annis (1974) (539 subjects) found an association between alcohol use in parents and in children as well as an association between use of pain killers by parents and by children.[48] However, in this study, parental use of barbiturates was not associated with increased barbiturate use in children. In all of these studies, predominant use of multiple types of drugs including alcohol were found to be transmitted from parents to children.

In a study of 6,447 high school students in Toronto in 1969, those students who had more marijuana and LSD use than expected had parents who used both alcohol and tobacco. The study did not inquire about parental use of psychoactive drugs such as tranquilizers, barbiturates, and stimulants. In a follow-up study of these students there was a positive association between reported drug use of parents and their adolescents. This relationship held for parental use of psychoactive drugs, tranquilizers, barbiturates, and stimulants, and for alcohol and tobacco on the one hand and for adolescent use of psychoactive and illicit hallucinogens on the other. Parents who were reported as frequent users of a psychoactive drug much more often had children who were using a hallucinogenic or psychoactive drug than parents who did not use these drugs. The relationship was very close when both parent and child were using the same drug (i.e., tranquilizers, barbiturates, or stimulants).[49]

In a study of 305 subjects with drug and/or alcohol abuse collected over a one-year period, a positive family history of alcohol abuse in first-degree relatives was found in 60% of the subjects and of drug abuse in 31% of the subjects. Significance was found for specificity; probands who were diagnosed as drug abusers were more likely to have a family history of drug abuse. Of the probands who had drug abuse, 18.5% had a positive first-degree family history of drug abuse only and 26% had a positive first-degree family history for both drug and alcohol abuse. Of the probands who had alcohol abuse only, 3% had a first degree family history positive for drugs only, and 14% had a positive family history for both drugs and alcohol. The relationship between drug abuse in parents and drug abuse in probands had the highest ratio, and was more impressive than the relationship between alcohol abuse in parents and drug abuse in probands. In this study, 82% (251) were male and 18% (54) were female, and of importance is that in the majority of subjects, 58% (177) were multiple drug addicts who met *DSM-III* criteria for both alcohol and drug abuse/dependence and not pure "drug abusers/dependents." Thirty-five percent (97) met criteria for alcohol abuse/dependence and 9% (27) met criteria for only nonalcoholic drug abuse/dependence.[50] Therefore, considerable overlap did exist between drug and alcohol abuse for probands and family members. Moreover, the rate of exposure to drugs in older family members such as parents was lower than that for the younger probands who have been exposed to nonalcoholic drugs at a higher rate. In interviews of 32 alcoholics, 72 opiate addicts, and 42 alcoholic opiate addicts, to a significant extent alcoholism tended to cluster in families whereas alcoholism and opiate abuse did not occur in the same families significantly more or less often than expected by chance alone using the contingency chi-square analysis.[51] It is important to note that overlap of alcoholism and opiate addiction did exist between relatives and probands, however, and that the lower rate of opiate addiction among alcoholic parents may have been due to the low rate of exposure to opiates in this generation. Additionally, a more recent study examining this hypothesis failed to find specific intergenerational transmission of opiate use from parents to offspring independent of alcohol dependence.[52]

A recent study of younger drug addicts showed familial history of drug abuse in 350 inpatients admitted for drug abuse in which 50% were opiate addicts, 33% were cocaine addicts and the remainder (17%) were sedative/hypnotic addicts. The rate of familial drug abuse corresponded to the proband's drug of choice, from 16% of male relatives of cocaine addicts to 2% of male relatives of sedative/hypnotic addicts. In support of a common familial transmission of drug and alcohol abuse is that the rate of alcoholism was the same across all proband groups regardless of drug type, indicating a high association of familial alcoholism and drug abuse in the proband.[53] Further support for a common transmission is a study of 41 male veterans that found an association between family history status of alcohol and drug dependence. Family history status did not discriminate onset of type of drug or alcohol abuse, i.e., "pure" alcohol abuse versus mixed alcohol and drug abuse. Two-thirds of the subjects were combined drug and alcohol abusers, while only one-third met criteria for pure alcohol abuse or dependence. Thus, the distribution of alcohol or drug abuse in the proband was not related to the family history status.[54]

CONCLUSIONS

The high prevalence of combined drug and alcohol use and addiction in drug addicts and alcoholics further supports mutual determinants of these disorders. Animal studies tend to support an individual and combined genetic vulnerability to drugs and alcohol.[2,3,4] Environment continues to play a major role in determining exposure to drugs and alcohol, particularly as seen in the widespread use of a variety of drugs and alcohol in recent decades.

Neurochemical models are being developed that accommodate a common biological substrate for drug and alcohol addiction. Animal and human studies have identified interactive integrated brain mechanisms that are activated by various drugs and alcohol and play major roles in the onset and sustenance of drug/alcohol addictions.[2,3,4]

The implications for treatment strategies are clear. Therapies directed at a single addiction will have limited efficacy as many drug addicts and alcoholics seeking treatment are multiply addicted. Moreover, the prognosis for the development of other drug and alcohol addictions in a particular individual addicted to a single drug is greatly influenced by the generalized vulnerability to drugs and alcohol.

REFERENCES

1. Miller NS, Gold MS. A neuroanatomical and neurochemical approach to drug and alcohol addiction: clinical and research considerations. In: Miller NS, ed. Comprehensive handbook of drug and alcohol addiction. New York: Marcel Dekker, 1991.

2. Wise RA. The brain and reward. In: Liebman JM, Cooper SJ, eds. The neuropharmacological basis of reward. Oxford University Press, 1989.

3. Trachtenberg MC, Blum K. Alcohol and opioid peptides: neuropharmacological rationale for physical cravings. Am J Drug Alcohol Abuse. 1987; 13(3): 365-72.

4. Blum K. A commentary on neurotransmitter restoration as a common mode of treatment for alcohol, cocaine and opiate abuse. Integr Psychiatry. 1989; 6:199-204.

5. Collins AC, Marks MJ. Progress towards the development of animal models of smoking-related behaviors. J Addict Dis. 1991; 10(1/2):109-126.

6. Pomerleau OF. Individual differences in sensitivity to nicotine: implications for genetic research on nicotine dependence. Behav Genet. 1995; 25(2): 161-177.

7. Gorelick DA. Serotonin uptake blockers and the treatment of alcoholism. In: Galanter MS, ed. Recent developments in alcoholism. New York: Plenum Press, 1988.

8. Kalivas PW, Widerlöv E, Stanley D, Breese G, Prange AJ. Enkephalin action on the mesolimbic system: a dopamine-dependent and dopamine-independent increase in locomotor activity. J Pharmacol Exp Ther. 1983; 227:229-37.

9. Miller NS, Gold MS. Research approaches to inheritance of alcoholism. J Subst Abuse Treat. 1988; 9(3):157-63.

10. Grant BF, Harford TC. Concurrent and simultaneous use of alcohol with cocaine: results of a national survey. Drug Alcohol Depend. 1990; 25:97-104.

11. Grant BF, Harford TC. Concurrent and simultaneous use of alcohol with sedatives and with tranquilizers: results of a national survey. J Subst Abuse Treat. 1990; 2:1-14.

12. Jekel JF, Allen DF. Trends in drug use in the mid-1980s. Yale J Biol Med. 1987; 60:45-52.

13. Kaufman E. The relationship of alcoholism and alcohol abuse to the abuse of other drugs. Am J Drug Alcohol Abuse. 1982; 9(1):1-17.

14. Needle R, Su S, Doherty W, Lavee Y, Brown P. Familial, interpersonal, and intrapersonal correlates of drug use: a longitudinal comparison of adolescents in treatment, drug-using adolescents not in treatment, and non-drug-using adolescents. Int J Addict. 1988; 23(12):1211-40.

15. Kandel DB, Raveis VH. Cessation of illicit drug use in young adulthood. Arch Gen Psychiatry. 1989; 46:409-16.

16. Freed EX. Drug abuse by alcoholics: a review. Int J Addict. 1973; 8:451-73.

17. Miller NS, Gold MS, eds. Alcohol. New York: Plenum Press, 1991.

18. Kosten TR, Rounsaville BJ, Babor TF, Spitzer RL, Williams JBW. Substance-use disorders in DSM-III-R. Br J Psychiatry. 1987; 151:834-43.

19. Miller NS, Millman RB, Keskinen S. Outcome at six and twelve months post inpatient treatment for cocaine and alcohol dependence. Adv Alcohol Subst Abuse. 1990; 9(3/4):101-20.

20. Miller NS. Special problems of the alcohol and multiple-drug dependent: clinical interactions and detoxification. In: Frances RJ, Miller SI, eds. Clinical textbook of addictive disorders. New York: Guilford Press, 1991.

21. Schmitz J, DeJong J, Garnett D, Moore V, Waxman R, Linnoila M, Roy A, Lamparski D. Substance abuse among subjects seeking treatment for alcoholism. (Letter to the Editor). Arch Gen Psychiatry. 1991; 48:182-83.

22. Schnoll SH, Karrigan J, Kitchen SB, et al. Characteristics of cocaine abusers presenting for treatment. NIDA Res Monogr. 1985; 85:171-81.

23. Miller NS, Millman RB, Keskinen S. The diagnosis of alcohol, cocaine, and other drug dependence in an inpatient treatment population. J Subst Abuse Treat. 1989; 6:37-40.

24. Miller NS. Special problems of the alcohol and multiple-drug dependent: clinical interactions and detoxification. In: Frances RJ, Miller SI, eds. Clinical textbook of addictive disorders. New York: The Guilford Press, 1991:194-218.

25. Goodwin DW. Alcoholism and genetics: the sins of our fathers. Arch Gen Psychiatry. 1985; 42:171-4.

26. Svikis DS, Pickens RW. Methodological issues in family, adoption, and twin research. NIDA Res Monogr. 1988; 89:120-33.

27. Cloninger CR. Etiologic factors in substance abuse: an adoption study perspective. NIDA Res Monogr. 1988; 89:52-72.

28. Cadoret RJ, O'Gorman TW, Troughton E, Heywood E. Alcoholism and antisocial personality: Interrelationships, genetic and environmental factors. Arch Gen Psychiatry. 1984; 42:161-167.

29. Goodwin DW, Schulsinger F, Moller N, Hermansen L, Winokur G, Guze SB. Drinking problems in adopted and nonadopted sons of alcoholics. Arch Gen Psychiatry. 1974; 31:164-169.

30. Bohman M. Some genetic aspects of alcoholism and criminality: A population of adoptees. Arch Gen Psychiatry. 1978; 35:269-276.

31. Bohman M, Sigvardsson S, Cloninger R. Maternal inheritance of alcohol abuse: Cross-fostering analysis of adopted women. Arch Gen Psychiatry. 1981; 38:965-969.

32. Cadoret RJ, Troughton E, O'Gorman TW, Heywood E. An adoption study of genetic and environmental factors in drug abuse. Arch Gen Psychiatry. 1986; 43:1131-6.

33. Pickens RW, Svikis DS, McGue M. Heterogeneity in the inheritance of alcoholism: a study of male and female twins. Arch Gen Psychiatry. 1991; 48:19-28.

34. Kendler KS, Neale MC, Heath AC, Phil D, Kessler RC, Eaves LT. A twin study of alcoholism in women. Am J Psychiatry. 1984; 151(5):707-15.

35. Frances RJ, Timm S, Bucky S. Studies of familial and non-familial alcoholism. I. Demographic studies. Arch Gen Psychiatry. 1980; 37:564-6.

36. Cotton NS. The familial incidence of alcoholism. J Stud Alcohol. 1979; 40(1):89-116.

37. Miller NS, Gold MS. Cocaine and alcoholism: distinct or part of a spectrum. Psychiatr Ann. 1988; 18(9):538-9.

38. Jones RW. Alcoholism among relatives of alcoholic patients. Q J Stud Alcohol. 1972; 33:810-813.

39. Miller NS, Gold MS, Belkin BM, Klahr AL. The diagnosis of alcohol and cannabis dependence in cocaine dependents and alcohol dependence in their families. Br J Addict. 1989; 84:1491-8.

40. Kosten TR, Rounsaville BJ, Kleber HD. Parental alcoholism in opioid addicts. J Nerv Ment Dis. 1987; 173(8):461-8.

41. Gfoerer J. Correlation between drug use by teenagers and drug use by older family members. Am J Drug Alcohol Abuse. 1987; 13(1/2):95-108.

42. Kandel DB, Kessler RC, Marguiles RZ. Antecedents of adolescent initiation into stages of drug use: a development analysis. J Adolesc Health. 1978; 7:13-40.

43. Tec N. Parent-child drug abuse: generational continuity or adolescent deviancy? Adolescence. 1974; 9:351-4.

44. Pandina RJ, Johnson V. Familial drinking history as a predictor of alcohol and drug consumption among adolescent children. J Stud Alcohol. 1989; 50(3): 245-53.

45. Pandina RJ, Johnson V. Serious alcohol and drug problems among adolescents with a family history of alcoholism. J Stud Alcohol. 1990; 51(3):278-282.

46. Scherer SE, Mukherjee BN. "Moderate" and hard drug users among college students: a study of their drug use patterns and characteristics. Br J Addict. 1971; 66:315-28.

47. Fawzy FI, Coombs RH, Gerber B. Generational continuity in the use of substances: the impact of parental substance use on adolescent substance abuse. Addict Behav. 1983; 8:109-14.

48. Annis HM. Patterns of intrafamilial drug use. Br J Addict. 1974; 69:361-9.

49. Smart RG, Fejer D. Drug use among adolescents and their parents: closing the generation gap in mood modification. J Abnorm Psychol. 1972; 79(2):153-60.

50. Meller WH, Rinehart R, Cadoret RJ, Troughton E. Specific familial transmission in substance abuse. Int J Addict. 1988; 23(10):1029-39.

51. Hill SY, Cloninger CR, Ayre FR. Independent familial transmission of alcoholism and opiate abuse. Alcohol Clin Exp Res. 1977; 1:335-42.

52. Rounsaville BJ, Kosten TR, Weissman MM, Prusoff B, Pauls D, Anton SF, Merikangas K. Psychiatric disorders in relatives of probands with opiate addiction. Arch Gen Psychiatry. 1991; 48(1):33-42.

53. Mirin SM, Weiss RD, Griffin ML, Michael JL. Psychopathology in drug abusers and their families. Compr Psychiatry. 1991; 32(1):36-51.

54. Moss HB. Psychopathy, aggression, and family history in male veteran substance abuse patients: a factor analytic study. Addict Behav. 1989; 14:565-70.

Psychopharmacotherapy for Addictive and Comorbid Disorders: Current Studies

Bradley M. Pechter, MD
Norman S. Miller, MD

SUMMARY. Proper diagnosis of comorbid disorders is crucial in treatment planning for the dually diagnosed. Since psychoactive substance use can obfuscate the diagnosis, special care must be taken to exclude organically based syndromes. Adequate periods of abstinence should first be achieved and subsequently the patient re-examined for residual symptoms compatible with a nonaddictive, nonsubstance-induced psychiatric disorder.

The integration of concurrent treatment of both the mental and the addictive disorders appears to be the best approach for treatment of comorbid psychiatric and addictive disorders. An abstinence-based model that typically utilizes a 12-step group therapy is often employed for the addictive illnesses. Other forms of psychosocial therapies such as case managers are being used as well.

Presently, physicians' prescribing practices for comorbid addicted patients are based on traditional approaches to use of medications in psychiatric patients, and their attitudes towards addictive disorders

Bradley M. Pechter is Assistant Professor of Psychiatry and Norman S. Miller is Associate Professor of Psychiatry and Neurology at the University of Illinois at Chicago, Chicago, IL.

Address correspondence to: Norman S. Miller, MD, The University of Illinois at Chicago, Department of Psychiatry (M/C 913), 912 South Wood Street, Chicago, IL 60612-7327.

[Haworth co-indexing entry note]: "Psychopharmacotherapy for Addictive and Comorbid Disorders: Current Studies." Pechter, Bradley M., and Norman S. Miller. Co-published simultaneously in *Journal of Addictive Diseases* (The Haworth Medical Press, an imprint of The Haworth Press, Inc.) Vol. 16, No. 4, 1997, pp. 23-40; and: *The Integration of Pharmacological and Nonpharmacological Treatments in Drug/Alcohol Addictions* (ed: Norman S. Miller, and Barry Stimmel) The Haworth Medical Press, an imprint of The Haworth Press, Inc., 1997, pp. 23-40. Single or multiple copies of this article are available for a fee from The Haworth Document Delivery Service [1-800-342-9678, 9:00 a.m. - 5:00 p.m. (EST). E-mail address: getinfo@haworth.com].

may play a significant role in determining the overall success of treatment. *[Article copies available for a fee from The Haworth Document Delivery Service: 1-800-342-9678. E-mail address: getinfo@haworth.com]*

INTRODUCTION

As Miller and Gold report, studies have supported a neurochemical origin for the addictive use of alcohol and other drugs through reinforcement centers in the limbic system.[1] The ventral tegmental area (VTA) in the midbrain, with its projections to the nucleus accumbens (NA) in the forebrain, is the mesolimbic pathway that is identified with compulsive use of drugs/alcohol. Dopamine (DA), the principal neurotransmitter involved, is contained in neurons in the VTA and is released in synapses in the NA. Other neurotransmitters such as serotonin (5-HT), gamma-aminobutyric acid (GABA), and norepinephrine (NE) appear to also contribute significantly by interacting with DA in the VTA.[2-4] Neuropeptides and enkephalins synapse on opiate receptors in DA neurons in the VTA. Of importance, these same neuroanatomical areas and their relevant neurotransmitters have also been implicated in the pathogenesis of several mental disorders, such as schizophrenia and bipolar disorders, and may share common vulnerability with addictive illness. Thus, medications that impact upon these neurochemical systems may not only have effects on the psychiatric disorder but also on the concurrent addictive disorders.

Miller and Gold argue that "pharmacological treatments for addictive disorders that suppress the appetitive, instinctual, or motivational drive states in the limbic system will likely have the most specific action on addictive disorders. The substrate for reinforcement of drug use utilizes the mesolimbic pathways, where neurotransmitter systems such as serotonin, dopamine, enkephalin, GABA, and norepinephrine interact. The development of medications could be aimed at these target structures as the primary generators of addictive drug and alcohol use."[1]

Indeed, abundant research efforts are focusing on these systems. Myers, in a review of these efforts in animal models of alcoholism, concurs that opioid, dopaminergic, and serotonergic systems are the most crucial ones modulating experimental alcoholism.[5] He reports that experimental medications such as amperozide modulate dopaminergic and serotonergic pathways while demonstrating some antipsychotic, antidepressant, anxiolytic, and "alcoholytic" actions. These experimental explorations meld with newer and established treatments for psychosis, depression, and anxiety, perhaps also establishing the foundation for treatment of the dually diagnosed. Conceivably, future drug therapies may effectively and efficiently treat both conditions simultaneously.

Despite the complexities inherent in treating the dually diagnosed, research and clinical practice must move forward to meet other challenges. Even as we begin to answer important questions in the area of dual diagnosis, questions about the treatment of "triple" diagnosis and beyond are emerging. For example, those with addiction, HIV or AIDS, and a concurrent mental disorder are a natural extension of a "simple" dual-diagnosis paradigm.[6] Other scenarios might include mental retardation complicated by a psychiatric plus addictive illness and should also be the focus of future clinical research. Presently, there is a clear need for further controlled studies of medications to treat the dually diagnosed.

Given our present state of knowledge, we have developed reasonable treatment strategies, as outlined in Figures 1-3. These figures address the treatment of psychotic, affective, and severe anxiety disorders complicated by alcohol or stimulant dependence (or the combination). We have chosen these substances, in part, to represent the most commonly encountered dual-diagnosis scenarios.

Proper diagnosis of comorbid disorders is crucial in treatment planning for the dually diagnosed. Since psychoactive substance use can obfuscate the diagnosis, special care must be taken to exclude organically based syndromes. Adequate periods of abstinence should first be achieved and subsequently the patient re-examined for residual symptoms compatible with a non-addictive, non-substance-induced psychiatric disorder.

PSYCHOPHARMACOTHERAPY FOR SPECIFIC DISORDERS

Medications

In general, clinicians tend to use pharmacological agents for the primary psychiatric disorder while integrating a concurrent non-

FIGURE 1. Treatment strategy for psychosis.

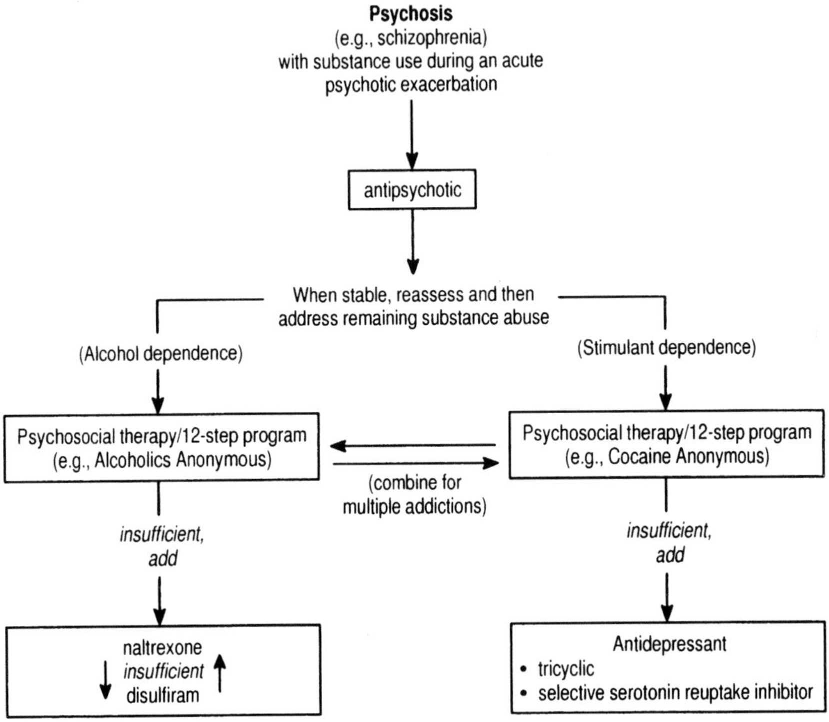

pharmacological treatment strategy for the addiction problem.[7,8] The integrated treatment of both the mental and the addictive disorders appears to be the best approach for treatment of comorbid addictive and other psychiatric diagnoses.[4,9] For the addiction, an abstinence-based model that typically utilizes a 12-step-based group therapy is most often employed.[10] Presently, physicians' prescribing practices for comorbid addicted patients are based on traditional approaches to the use of medications in psychiatric patients, and their attitudes towards addictive disorders may play a significant role in determining the treatment strategy.[8]

The use of psychotropic medication without simultaneous attention to the addictive disorder is not likely to produce the desired results for the addiction or the concurrent psychiatric condition. There are also some relative contraindications to using certain psy-

FIGURE 2. Treatment strategy for major depression.

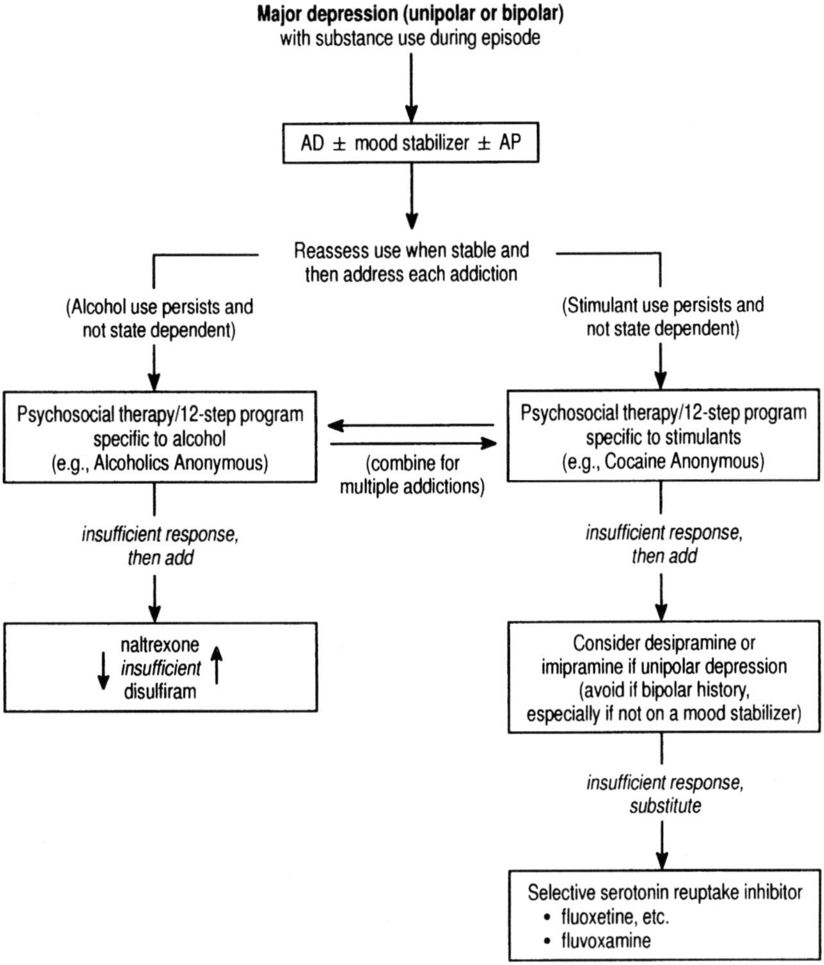

chotropics in the addicted with other psychiatric disorders. For example, benzodiazepines, despite their benefit, are also subject to addictive use and acute and chronic use in these patients with a history of addictive disorders. In addition, antidepressants and antipsychotics with high anticholinergic properties should be used conservatively because of their potential for misuse and addictive use.

FIGURE 3. Treatment strategy for anxiety disorders.

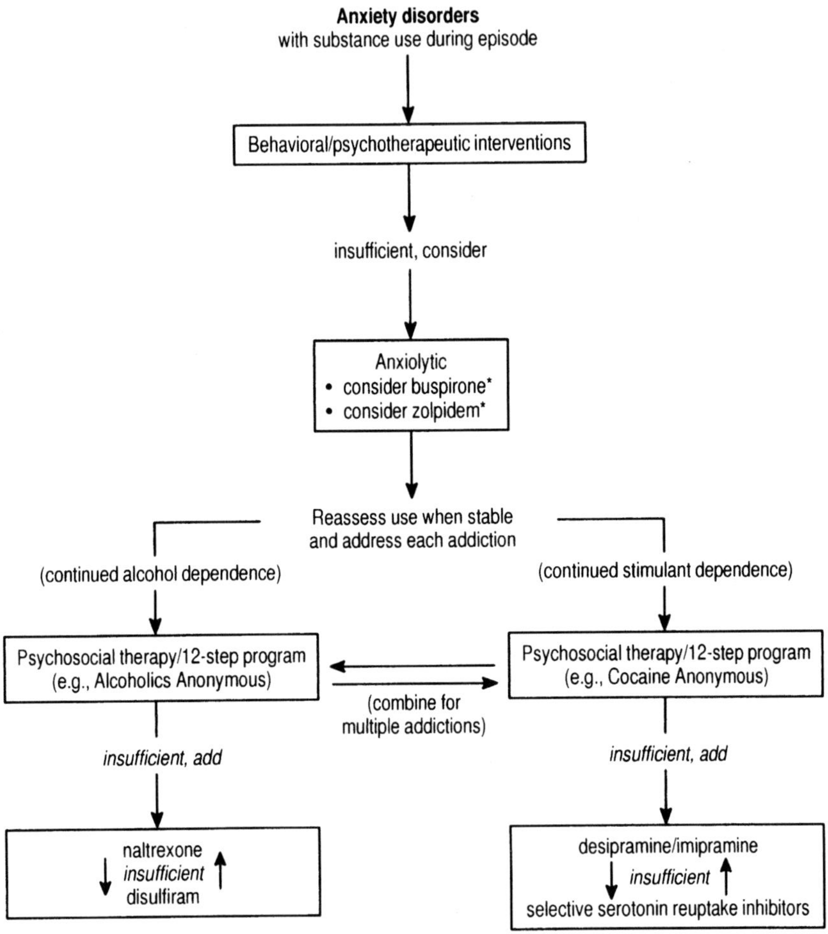

* These are nonaddictive, nonbenzodiazepine agents. Zolpidem may be especially effective with insomnia.

Mood Disorders

Unipolar Depression

While depression in the dually diagnosed is a frequently studied problem, there can be considerable difficulty in diagnosing a true, independent major depressive episode in the presence of active concurrent addiction.[11] Often, a period of abstinence is necessary; but it is unclear as to the minimum time necessary before attempting to finalize the diagnosis. For example, the DSM-IV requires that depressive symptoms "persist for a substantial period of time (e.g., about a month)" after acute withdrawal or intoxication to be called substance-induced mood disorder.[12] Some transitory depressive symptoms are common in the first few weeks of abstinence after a prolonged period of substance use. This may be a part of the withdrawal or a reaction to the patient's "hitting bottom." There is ample evidence that while alcoholism and depression are often associated, they may also present as distinct entities and not different presentations of identical processes.[13] As a result, there is often an overlapping of common symptoms, which makes proper diagnosis much more difficult.

Clinical studies in depressed alcoholics give some suggestions of the course of treatments. Brown and co-workers demonstrated that those male patients in their sample who were dually diagnosed with alcohol dependence and a mood disorder did not demonstrate more severe depressive symptoms or a slower recovery than their counterparts with either diagnosis alone.[14] There is evidence from another study that depression upon acute inpatient admission in schizophrenic alcoholics resolves along the same timeframe as does depression in non-dually diagnosed alcoholics.[15] If supported and broadened by further investigation, this finding would simplify treatment strategies by including the dually diagnosed *into established trends for mainstream addiction treatment.*

Tricyclic Antidepressants (TCAs). The role of tricyclics for depressed alcoholics has usually been limited to the period of acute withdrawal and not for longer term maintenance. Other methodological problems with studies in this area include: relative inattention to different subtypes of depression; inadequate use of therapeutic drug monitoring; and failure to monitor both mood and drinking behavior in response to treatment.[16]

Despite these design flaws, many of the studies support the beneficial effects of tricyclic antidepressants in the treatment of depression associated with alcohol withdrawal. These benefits, however, do not exceed those of placebo after 3 weeks and thus may have only limited application to the "real world" of clinical practice.

Of the antidepressants presently available, imipramine is the most extensively studied. A recent trial assessing this agent's effectiveness for alcoholism with comorbid depression in methadone-maintenance patients had certain advantages over its predecessors, including: lifetime histories to make diagnoses of depression (thus avoiding transient depressive effects of alcohol); a double-blind design during the second phase of the study; and adequacy of dosing as monitored by plasma levels.[17]

Unfortunately, the criteria for response are incomplete, but the authors report that of 60 alcoholics with major depression who completed an initial 12-week *open-label* trial of imipramine, 27 (45%) responded, showing improvement in both mood (post-treatment Hamilton Depression Rating Scale score = 3; SD = 3) and drinking behavior (30% achieving abstinence and another 15% at a "much reduced level"). These response rates were further enhanced after dosage increases or treatment with disulfiram. Patients who improved with imipramine in the initial open trial were then randomized into a subsequent 6-month double-blind maintenance phase. During this phase, 7 of 10 (70%) relapsed on placebo in contrast to only 4 of 13 (31%) on imipramine. Although the sample sizes were small, the authors believed that this represented a significant improvement for those on medication in a common dual-diagnosis scenario.

Support for the efficacy of imipramine in treating depression in dual diagnosis was also found in one *open-label* trial of depressed patients in a methadone maintenance program.[18] The results of this preliminary evaluation suggested that both mood and illicit drug use improved.

Desipramine versus placebo was studied in a 12-week, double-blind design comparing depressed to non-depressed cocaine-dependent methadone-maintenance patients.[19] Here, desipramine led to less overall cocaine use, and by week 10 the medicated depressed patients still in treatment had a 68% reduction in cocaine craving and a 96% reduction in cocaine use compared with their counterparts in the placebo group. By the final 12 weeks of the trial, 0% of urine toxicology screens were cocaine-free for depressed patients in the placebo group compared with 33% for the depressed patients on desipramine. The percentage of cocaine-free screens was 50% over the same period when only study completers were included. Despite the small sample size this study supports the efficacy of desipramine as an adjunctive therapy for cocaine addiction.

The Selective Serotonin Reuptake Inhibitors (SSRIs). New possibilities exist with the emergence of the selective serotonin reuptake inhibitors. Basic studies in animals which used these agents have substantiated a decrease in alcohol preference and consumption, while non-specific monoamine uptake blockers (e.g., amitriptyline, doxepin) have not.[20] Gorelick reported evidence, using animal models of spontaneous alcohol consumption, that increased brain serotonin activity tended to decrease alcohol preference and consumption. Extrapolating these results from the laboratory to the clinical arena, Gorelick and Paredes then studied the effect of fluoxetine on alcohol consumption in 20 males with chronic dependence.[21] After a 28-day double-blind, placebo-controlled period, they found that the fluoxetine group had a 14% lower alcohol intake, primarily during the first week. The beneficial effect was associated with a lower proportion of requests as well as less craving for alcohol. Unfortunately, and similar to the imipramine outcomes, these investigators did not find a significant effect in later weeks (i.e., virtually no differences in scores on the Hamilton Depression and Anxiety Scales or the abridged Hopkins Symptom Checklist (SCL-58)).

While the SSRIs' mechanism of action in treating alcoholism remains unclear, Gorelick postulates that it is not due to motor inhibition or general sedation. Rather, he believes it may be "related to decreased appetite and food intake or a conditioned taste aversion mediated by increased brain serotonin activity."[21]

Several outpatient studies of SSRIs used in early-stage problem drinkers and chronic alcoholics have also supported this trend by demonstrating reductions in various parameters used to measure drinking over variable time frames.[22-24]

Currently, we are aware of no studies using the SSRIs that specifically examine treatment in the dually diagnosed patient. In fact, the avoidance of significant depressive symptoms in subjects involved in these early studies was important to their design to avoid contaminating the outcome due to the specific antidepressant action of these agents. Thus, the need for trials with this class of antidepressants in the dually diagnosed population is an important next step, particularly in light of the positive findings with imipramine. Analogous to the treatment of depression, the SSRIs may offer similar benefits with considerably less risk as compared to the TCAs.

Bipolar Disorder

There is a high incidence of comorbid addiction in bipolar disorder. Clinical and epidemiological studies show between 15%-40% of bipolar patients are addicted to alcohol and/or other drugs.[25] Data on the bipolar population shows that concurrent substance users had an earlier age of onset; were hospitalized twice as often for mood problems; were four times more likely to have other Axis I disorders; and were twice as likely to have dysphoric mania than their non-substance abusing counterparts.[26] Diagnosis and treatment of this population is further complicated by the fact that many addictive substances produce manic-like symptoms. Indeed, even relatively benign drugs frequently used in the general population, such as caffeine and ephedrine, may induce or exacerbate manic episodes in those who are predisposed. In general, all mood-stabilizing agents used for the dually diagnosed can at least facilitate treatment of the psychiatric and the addictive disorders by stabilizing the patient and promoting more appropriate participation in treatment.

Lithium, still considered by many the treatment of choice for bipolar disorder, has not fulfilled initial promise for the treatment of primary alcoholism with and without a concurrent affective disorder. Dorus and colleagues studied 457 male alcoholics in a VA collaborative study and found that lithium did not alter the use of alcohol in either depressed or non-depressed alcoholics.[27] Specifically, they reported abstinence in 38% of lithium-treated non-depressed alcoholics (compared with 28% of placebo controls) and 32% of lithium-treated depressed alcoholics (compared to 37% of their placebo controls). Fawcett et al., who studied 104 alcoholics in a double-blind, placebo-controlled design, report beneficial effects of lithium in this population, but they found that 19 of 51 (37%) patients given lithium and 22 of 53 (42%) patients on placebo were abstinent at the 6-month follow-up, with the numbers becoming even more similar at the 12-month follow-up.[28]

Although lithium no longer appears promising to treat alcohol dependence itself, it may yet have a place in pharmacotherapy of the overall affective syndrome. A small pilot study (N = 12) by Nagel et al. assessed lithium in a double-blind, placebo-controlled design focusing on recently (3 to 7 days before entry into study) detoxified alcoholics who manifested a syndrome resembling hypomania.[29] Symptoms consisted of elevated psychomotor activity, grandiosity, irritability, a heightened desire for social contact, loquaciousness, and sexual preoccupation. The severity of symptoms was significantly decreased by treatment with low-dose lithium carbonate (serum levels 0.3 to 0.5 meq/liter) but was not affected by placebo treatment.

Anticonvulsants such as divalproex sodium and carbamazepine are effective mood-stabilizing agents and have the added advantage of being useful in withdrawal states secondary to alcohol, benzodiazepines, and cocaine.[30,31] Since lithium may show some utility in certain dually diagnosed bipolar patients and the anticonvulsants attenuate several types of withdrawal syndromes, the latter agents may possibly emerge as effective and safe treatments for bipolar alcoholics.

Anxiety Related Disorders

Anxiety is a common complaint that invariably complicates addictive illnesses. Decker and Ries cite estimates of comorbid anxiety and alcohol syndromes, many substance-induced, ranging from 20 to 50%.[32-35] Patients with alcohol or drug dependence show a tendency to develop panic symptoms earlier, and it has been observed that repeated alcohol withdrawal mimics panic attacks in many individuals.[36,37] Finally, benzodiazepines, the primary pharmacologic treatment for these disorders, are themselves addictive and sometimes associated with anxiety syndromes, especially upon their discontinuation.[38]

There are presently few studies involving pharmacotherapy for co-existing anxiety and addictive disorders, but future investigations should consider buspirone, a non-benzodiazepine partial serotonin agonist with anxiolytic properties. This agent may be particularly valuable in treating the dually diagnosed because it is non-addicting. In this light, a placebo-controlled trial of buspirone in anxious alcoholics by Kranzler et al. indicated that this agent led to a greater likelihood of completing treatment, reduction of anxiety symptoms, a slower rate of heavy alcohol relapse, and more days of abstinence during the follow-up period.[39]

Psychotic Disorders

Schizophrenics have a high rate of substance-related disorders in epidemiological studies, i.e., 50-90%. Alcoholism and drug addiction in schizophrenics represents two concurrent diseases-addictive and chronic mental illness in the same individual. It is interesting that in their assessment of the literature Decker and Ries, as well as Smith and Hucker, found that no particular substance seems to be preferentially used by schizophrenic patients with addictions. And while they write that "there is little evidence that opiates contribute to increased psychosis," other substances are known to have some psychotogenic qualities such as paranoia and/or hallucinations that can be associated with alcohol, cocaine or amphetamines, cannabis, and LSD or hallucinogens.[12]

In the area of therapy, Bowers and Mazure reported the results from a study using fixed doses of haloperidol or perphenazine to treat psychotic patients with and without concurrent addiction.[40] They found that psychotic males with prior use of addictive substances had a poorer early response (first 10 days) to antipsychotics when compared to their counterparts who had no addictive use of substances. They hypothesized that such earlier drug use had contributed to increased psychosis and to relative antipsychotic refractoriness, perhaps mediated by dopaminergic mechanisms. While this study had several methodological disadvantages (e.g., not blinded, no random assignment, no significant drug washout period, possibly sub-optimal plasma levels, and short duration), it nonetheless suggests a diminished responsiveness to antipsychotics in the dual-diagnosis population. This initial drug refractoriness may have important clinical and theoretical significance that clearly needs further investigation and may discourage a cautious optimism in treatment of such patients.

In another study, patients with or without a history of addictive disorders attained similar improvements on clozapine.[41] In light of this study, as well as other observations, the authors hypothesize that clozapine may have a unique ability to decrease drug craving in schizophrenic patients who are dually diagnosed.

A third study reported that dually diagnosed schizophrenic patients show predominantly negative symptoms early in the course of their illness, which then progresses to a mixed (i.e., positive and negative symptoms) presentation.[42] This, the authors note, is in marked contrast to the usual course in schizophrenia, in which positive symptoms occur early in the course of illness and then recede as negative symptoms gain prominence. This observation may also have relevance for drug treatment strategies of dually diagnosed psychotic disorders.

Finally, desipramine was studied in a 12-week open-label design in 27 outpatient schizophrenic cocaine addicts who were also treated with appropriate antipsychotic regimens, relapse prevention, and social skills training programs.[43] The group receiving desipramine (100 to 150 mg/day) was more likely to complete the study, had fewer cocaine-positive urines, and had improved psychiatric symptoms during the study. While these results are consistent with the outcome in some studies using desipramine for cocaine addiction without psychiatric comorbidity, we note that there is disagreement in the literature regarding desipramine's effectiveness in reducing cocaine dependence.[19,44-46] To our knowledge, this is the only study using antidepressants in the literature on dually diagnosed psychotic patients.

Opiate Antagonists in Schizophrenic Disorders

Psychiatric Disorders with Comorbid Alcohol Problems

As yet, no naltrexone studies have focused on schizophrenic or bipolar alcoholics. The findings of the trials already mentioned, as well as the possible benefits of opiate antagonists in treating symptoms of schizophrenia or bipolar disorder without alcohol abuse, however, warrant studies in these difficult-to-treat populations.[47,48]

There are approximately 25 studies, most of them single or double-blind, that have investigated the effects of naloxone or naltrexone on hallucinations in schizophrenic patients. While about one-third found that these drugs decreased hallucinations, two-thirds failed to find such an effect. Of the two studies that examined the effects of naltrexone in mania, one found an attenuation of symptoms and the other did not.[49,50]

Most of this literature studied the effects of one injection of naltrexone versus one injection of placebo to see whether hallucinations and delusions decreased. While one open naltrexone study that ran for several weeks reported benefit in many schizophrenic patients, several others have not.[51-56] Since these studies generally investigated naltrexone alone, its role as an adjunctive therapy with antipsychotics has not been adequately addressed. Given that there is no evidence to suggest that naltrexone is deleterious in the treatment of psychiatric disorders, we feel it is important to determine if it might improve hallucinations and delusions when used to augment standard antipsychotic drug therapy.

In summary, we believe naltrexone is an especially promising agent in the pharmacotherapy of coexisting psychiatric and addictive disorders. To this end we are presently conducting a double-blind, placebo-controlled study examining its effectiveness in alcoholics also diagnosed with major psychotic or mood disorders, especially when combined with effective psychosocial interventions.

Disulfiram in Schizophrenics. Disulfiram is sometimes quite helpful as an adjunct to nonpharmacological treatments for alcoholism. While it has the potential to worsen psychosis, Kofoed cautions that these findings are based upon untreated chronic patients given high doses.[57,58]

Kofoed et al. used disulfiram with a small number of dually diagnosed psychotic and alcohol-dependent patients after they were stabilized on appropriate antipsychotic medications. They found that compliance with disulfiram therapy in their dual-diagnosis group was as good as in primary alcoholic outpatients. They also reported no particular problems, concluding that disulfiram seemed less of a risk than continued alcohol misuse.[59,60]

Methadone in Schizophrenics. We are aware of no evidence demonstrating that methadone interferes with antipsychotic function. It is the opinion of one author, based upon a small trial, that methadone may have some inherent antipsychotic properties when used as an adjunct to standard antipsychotics.[61] For these reasons, we believe that psychosis itself is not a contraindication for an otherwise eligible patient to receive this drug for maintenance therapy of narcotic dependence. Furthermore, this agent may help stabilize patients sufficiently so they can participate in appropriate treatments for their dual-diagnosis problem.

CONCLUSION

The treatment of comorbid psychiatric and addictive disorders often involves the use of pharmacological agents. Addictive disorders commonly co-occur with psychiatric disorders, particularly, with chronic mental illnesses. Pharmacotherapies can be indispensable to the treatment of comorbid disorders whereas integration of psychotherapies for addictive disorders is essential.

REFERENCES

1. Miller NS, Gold MS. The psychiatrist's role in integrating pharmacological and nonpharmacological treatments for addictive disorders. Psychiatric Annals. 1992;22(8):436-40.

2. Gold MS, Miller NS. Seeking drugs/alcohol and avoiding withdrawal. Psychiatric Annals. 1992;22(8):430-5.

3. Miller NS, Gold MS. A neurochemical model for alcohol and drug addiction. J Psychoactive Drugs. 1993;25(2):121-8.

4. Miller NS. Issues in the diagnosis and treatment of comorbid addictive and other psychiatric disorders. Directions in Psychiatry. 1994;14(25):1-8.

5. Myers RD. New drugs for the treatment of experimental alcoholism. Alcohol. 1994;11(6):439-51.

6. Batki SL. Drug abuse, psychiatric disorders, and AIDS: Dual and triple diagnosis. West J Med. 1990;152(5):547-52.

7. Adelman SA, Fletcher KE, Bahnassi A, et al. The scale for treatment integration of the dually diagnosed (STIDD): An instrument for assessing intervention strategies in the pharmacotherapy of mentally ill substance abusers. Drug Alcohol Depend. 1991;27:35-42.

8. Adelman SA, Fletcher KE, Bahnassi A. Pharmacotherapeutic management strategies for mentally ill substance abusers. J Subst Abuse Treat. 1993;10:353-8.

9. Minkoff K. An integrated treatment model for dual diagnosis of psychosis and addiction. Hospital and Community Psychiatry. 1989;40:1031-6.

10. Roman PM. Inpatient alcohol and drug treatment: a national study of treatment centers. Executive Report. Institute for Behavioral Research, University of

Georgia. Supported by National Institute of Alcohol Abuse and Addiction. 1989; 1:22.

11. Dackis CA, Gold MS, Pottash ALC, et al. Evaluating depression in alcoholics. Psychiatry Res. 1986;17:105-9.

12. American Psychiatric Association: Diagnostic and statistical manual of mental disorders, 4th edition. Washington, D.C, American Psychiatric Association, 1994.

13. Merikangas KR, Leckman JF, Prusoff BA, et al. Familial transmission of depression and alcoholism. Arch Gen Psychiatry. 1985;42(4):367-72.

14. Brown SA, Inaba RK, Gillin JC, et al. Alcoholism and affective disorder: Clinical course of depressive symptoms. Am J Psychiatry. 1995;152:45-52.

15. Brady KT, Killeen T, Jarrell P. Depression in alcoholic schizophrenic patients. Am J Psychiatry. 1993;150:1255-6.

16. Ciraulo DA, Jaffe JH. Tricyclic antidepressants in the treatment of depression associated with alcoholism. J Clin Psychopharamacol. 1981;1:146-50.

17. Nunes EV, McGrath PJ, Quitkin FM, et al. Imipramine treatment of alcoholism with comorbid depression. Am J Psychiatry, 1993;150(6):963-5.

18. Nunes EV, Quitkin FM, Brady R, et al. Imipramine treatment of methadone maintenance patients with affective disorder and illicit drug use. Am J Psychiatry. 1991;148(5):667-9.

19. Ziedonis DM, Kosten TR. Depression as prognostic factor for pharmacological treatment of cocaine dependence. Psychopharmacol Bull. 1991;27:337-43.

20. Gorelick DA. Serotonin uptake blockers and the treatment of alcoholism. In Galanter M (ed): Recent developments in alcoholism, vol 7, pp. 267-81. New York, Plenum, 1989.

21. Gorelick DA, Paredes A. Effect of fluoxetine on alcohol consumption in male alcoholics. Alcohol Clin Exp Res. 1992;16(2):261-5.

22. Amit Z, Brown Z, Sutherland Z, et al. Reduction in alcohol intake in humans as a function of treatment with zimeldine: implications for treatment. In Naranjo CA, Sellers EM (eds): Research advances in new psychopharmacological treatments for alcoholism. Amsterdam, Excerpta Medica. 1985;189-98.

23. Naranjo CA, Sellers EM, Jullivan JT, et al. The serotonin uptake inhibitor citalopram attenuates ethanol intake. Clin Pharmacol Ther. 1987;41:266-74.

24. Naranjo CA, Sellers EM, Roach CA, et al. Zimeldine-induced variations in alcohol intake by non-depressed heavy drinkers. Clin Pharmacol Ther. 1984; 35:374-81.

25. Winokur G, Cook B, Liskow B, et al. Alcoholism in manic depressive (bipolar) patients. J Stud Alcohol. 1993;54:574-6.

26. Sonne SC, Brady KT, Morton WA. Substance abuse and bipolar affective disorder. J Nerv Ment Dis. 1994;182(6):349-52.

27. Dorus W, Ostrow DG, Anton R, et al. Lithium treatment of depressed and nondepressed alcoholics. JAMA. 1989;262:1646-52.

28. Fawcett J, Clark DC, Gibbons RD, et al. Evaluation of lithium therapy for alcoholism. J Clin Psychiatry. 1984;45:494-9.

29. Nagel K, Adler LE, Bell J, et al. Lithium carbonate and mood disorder in recently detoxified alcoholics: A double-blind, placebo-controlled pilot study. Alcohol Clin Exp Res. 1991;15(6):978-81.

30. Halikas J, Kuhn K, Carlsan G. The effect of carbamazepine on cocaine use. American Journal of Addictions. 1992;1(1):30-9.

31. Kosten TR, Gawin FH, Kosten TA, et al. Six month follow-up of short-term pharmacotherapy for cocaine dependence. American Journal of Addictions. 1992;1(1):40-9.

32. Decker KP, Ries RK. Differential diagnosis and psychopharmacology of dual disorders. Psychiatr Clin North Am. 1993;16(4):703-19.

33. Bowen RC, Cipywnyk D, D'Arcy C, et al. Alchoholism, anxiety disorders, and agoraphobia. Alcohol Clin Exp Res. 1984;8:48-50.

34. Smail P, Stockwell T, Canter S, et al. Alcohol dependence and phobic anxiety states I. A prevalence study. Br J Psychiatry. 1984;144:53-7.

35. Reich J, Chaudhry D. Personality of panic disorder alcohol abusers. J Nerv Ment Dis. 1987;175:224-8.

36. Starcevic V, Uhlenhuth EH, Kellner R, et al. Comorbidity in panic disorder:II. Chronology of appearance and pathogenic comorbidity. Psychiatry Res. 1993;46:285-93.

37. George DT, Nutt DJ, Dwyer BA, et al. Alcoholism and panic disorder: Is the comorbidity more than coincidence? Acta Psychiatr Scand. 1990;81:97-107.

38. Janicak PG, Davis JM, Preskorn SH, Ayd FJ Jr: Principles and practice of psychopharmacotherapy. Baltimore: Williams & Wilkins, 1993.

39. Kranzler HR, Burleson JA, Del Boca FK, et al. Buspirone treatment of anxious alcoholics: A placebo-controlled trial. Arch Gen Psychiatry. 1994;51:720-31.

40. Bowers MB, Mazure CM, Nelson JC, et al. Psychotogenic drug use and neuroleptic response. Schizophr Bull. 1990;16(1):81-5.

41. Buckley P, Thompson P, Way L, et al. Substance abuse among patients with treatment-resistant schizophrenia: Characteristics and implications for clozapine therapy. Am J Psychiatry. 1994;151(3):385-9.

42. Rosenthal RN, Hellerstein DJ, Miner CR. Positive and negative syndrome typology in schizophrenic patients with psychoactive substance use disorders. Compr Psychiatry. 1994;35(2):91-8.

43. Ziedonis D, Richardson T, Lee E, et al. Adjunctive desipramine in the treatment of cocaine abusing schizophrenics. Psychopharmacol Bull. 1992;28(3):309-14.

44. Gawin FH, Kleber HD, Byck R, et al. Desipramine facilitation in initial cocaine abstinence. Arch Gen Psychiatry. 1989;46:117-21.

45. Weddington WW, Brown BS, Haertzen CA, et al. Comparison of amantadine and desipramine combined with psychotherapy for treatment of cocaine dependence. Am J Drug Alcohol Abuse. 1991;17(2):137-52.

46. Arndt IO, McLellan AT, Dorozynsky L, et al. Desipramine treatment for cocaine dependence. J Nerv Ment Dis. 1994;182(3):151-6.

47. Berger P, Watson S, Akil H, et al. The effects of naloxone in chronic schizophrenia. Am J Psychiatry. 1981;138:913-5.

48. Watson SJ, Berger PA, Akil H, et al. Effects of naloxone in schizophrenia: Reduction in hallucinations in a subpopulation of subjects. Science. 1978;201:73-6.

49. Janowsky DS, Judd L, Huey L, et al. Naloxone effects on manic symptoms and growth-hormone levels. Lancet. 1978;i:320.

50. Verhoeven WMA, van Praag HM, de Jong JTVM. Use of naloxone in schizophrenic psychoses and manic syndromes. Neuropsychobiology. 1981;7:159-68.

51. Emrich HM, Cording C, Piree S, et al. Indication of an antipsychotic action of the opiate antagonist naloxone. Pharmakopsychiat. 1977;10:265-70.

52. Ragheb M, Berney S, Ban T. Naltrexone in chronic schizophrenia. Int Pharmacopsychiatry. 1980;15:1-5.

53. Simpson GM, Branchey MH, Lee JH. A trial of naltrexone in chronic schizophrenia. Curr Ther Res. 1977;22(6):909-13.

54. Mielke DH, Gaillant DM. An oral opiate antagonist in chronic schizophrenia: A pilot study. Am J Psychiatry. 1977;134:1430-1.

55. Gitlin M, Rosenblatt M. Possible withdrawal from endogenous opiates in schizophrenics. Am J Psychiatry. 1978;135(3):377-8.

56. Dysken MW, Davis JM (letter). Naloxone in amylobarbitone responsive catatonia. Br J Psychiatry. 1978;133:476-80.

57. Major LF, Lerner P, Ballenger JC, et al. Dopamine beta-hydroxylase in the cerebrospinal fluid: Relationship to disulfiram-induced psychosis. Biol Psychiatry. 1979;14:337-44.

58. Kofoed L. Outpatient vs. inpatient treatment for the chronically mentally ill with substance use disorders. J Addict Dis. 1993;12(3):123-37.

59. Kofoed L, Kania J, Walsh T, et al. Outpatient treatment of patients with substance abuse and coexisting psychiatric disorders. Am J Psychiatry. 1986;143: 867-72.

60. Kofoed LL. Chemical monitoring of disulfiram compliance: A study of alcoholic outpatients. Alcohol Clin Exp Res. 1987;11:481-5.

61. Britzer DA, Hartman N, Sweeney J, et al. Effect of methadone plus neuroleptics on treatment-resistant chronic paranoid schizophrenia. Am J Psychiatry. 1985;142:1106-7.

Integrating Treatments for Methamphetamine Abuse: A Psychosocial Perspective

Alice Huber, PhD
Walter Ling, MD
Steven Shoptaw, PhD
Vikas Gulati, BS
Paul Brethen, MA
Richard Rawson, PhD

SUMMARY. The recent West Coast experience with increased methamphetamine use is showing signs of spreading to other parts of the US. The risk of corresponding medical and psychosocial problems

---

Alice Huber, Walter Ling, Steven Shoptaw, Vikas Gulati, Paul Brethen, and Richard Rawson are affiliated with the Matrix Institute on Addictions. Alice Huber, Walter Ling, Steven Shoptaw and Richard Rawson are affiliated with the Los Angeles Addiction Treatment Research Center and the West Los Angeles VA Medication Development Research Unit. Walter Ling and Richard Rawson are also affiliated with the UCLA Alcoholism and Addiction Medicine Service.

Address correspondence to: Dr. Walter Ling, Los Angeles Addiction Treatment Research Center, 10350 Santa Monica Boulevard, Suite 340, Los Angeles, CA 90025.

This manuscript was supported by: a contract from the San Bernardino County Health Department to the Matrix Institute; NIDA grant (DA 06185) to Richard Rawson and Matrix Institute; NIDA grant for the LAATRC: Medications Development Research Center (DA 09260) to Walter Ling and Friends Research Institute; and, a NIDA Interagency Agreement (DA 50038) to Walter Ling and the West Los Angeles VA Medical Center.

[Haworth co-indexing entry note]: "Integrating Treatments for Methamphetamine Abuse: A Psychosocial Perspective." Huber, Alice et al. Co-published simultaneously in *Journal of Addictive Diseases* (The Haworth Medical Press, an imprint of The Haworth Press, Inc.) Vol. 16, No. 4, 1997, pp. 41-50; and: *The Integration of Pharmacological and Nonpharmacological Treatments in Drug/Alcohol Addictions* (ed: Norman S. Miller, and Barry Stimmel) The Haworth Medical Press, an imprint of The Haworth Press, Inc., 1997, pp. 41-50. Single or multiple copies of this article are available for a fee from The Haworth Document Delivery Service [1-800-342-9678, 9:00 a.m. - 5:00 p.m. (EST). E-mail address: getinfo@haworth.com].

has led to a call to action at the highest levels of government. The next few years will likely witness a substantial increase in treatment research on methamphetamine abuse/dependence, with particular emphasis on the development and application of novel pharmacotherapies. The evaluation of these agents presupposes that we understand the clinical syndrome resulting from chronic methamphetamine use. To establish a clear picture of the biological and psychological sequellae of methamphetamine use, we compare two cohorts (500 methamphetamine and 224 cocaine users) treated at the same outpatient clinic over the past nine years, using identical manualized treatments. The results suggest that while there are important differences in group characteristics and drug effects, the total response to treatment was quite comparable. *[Article copies available for a fee from The Haworth Document Delivery Service: 1-800-342-9678. E-mail address: getinfo@haworth.com]*

INTRODUCTION

Methamphetamine use in the western US is on the rise and the problems associated with its use are growing.[1] Methamphetamine-related visits to emergency rooms nationwide increased 256% from 1991 to 1994.[2] What has been until recently a "pocket" or regional problem suddenly threatens to become a serious national problem. Already signs of its spread are unmistakable. National media reports and national surveys[3] indicate that methamphetamine abuse is spreading in many major cities across the country. Moreover, some users (e.g., gay and bisexual men) engage in highly risky sexual activities under the influence of methamphetamine,[4] which has significant implications regarding HIV transmission.

As a result of the growing number of methamphetamine abusers, there has been considerable interest recently in developing integrated pharmacological and psychosocial treatments for methamphetamine abuse/dependence. The working models employed thus far have been borrowed largely from the cocaine experience of the 1980's. In order to gain an understanding of the clinical issues that need to be addressed in the treatment of methamphetamine abuse/dependence, it may be instructive to examine the similarities and differences between methamphetamine and cocaine users and their relative response to pharmacological and non-pharmacological treatments.

The recent explosion of attention given to methamphetamine

abuse in this country is likely to herald in a wave of research aimed at testing many different psychotropic treatment agents. As the pharmacotherapy research agenda for methamphetamine treatments is established, it would be helpful to know how methamphetamine users respond to psychosocial protocols. How should the effects of pharmacotherapies be assessed vis a vis treatment response to psychosocial protocols? Can the comparative treatment experience of methamphetamine and cocaine users to psychosocial treatment provide useful information about the nature of methamphetamine users' response to treatment medications? The lack of baseline nonpharmacological treatment response rate has compounded the interpretation of cocaine pharmacotherapeutic interventions in the past.[5] Therefore, an opportunity to compare the treatment experiences of a group of methamphetamine and cocaine abusers in a standardized psychosocial program should provide some background information for a more adequate explanation of pharmacotherapeutic responses. This report compares the baseline characteristics and treatment experiences of more than 700 methamphetamine and cocaine abusers treated at the Matrix clinic in Rancho Cucamonga, California.

METHOD

Clinic. The Matrix clinic is located in Rancho Cucamonga, a rural community approximately 45 miles east of Los Angeles. The clinic was established in 1985 to provide drug-free treatment for 150 alcohol- and drug-abusing persons annually. Although all types of dependence are treated, stimulant abuse treatment, and more specifically, methamphetamine treatment, is by far the predominant focus. This area has had a serious methamphetamine problem for years, and numerous indicators of problem levels of use in the county continue to rise.[6]

Sample. We completed an extensive review of the clinical charts for all stimulant-using individuals who sought treatment at the clinic between 1988 and 1995. For individuals with multiple treatment episodes, only data from the initial episode were included. The final sample comprised 500 methamphetamine- and 224 cocaine-abusing persons.

Measures. Throughout the period covered by the study, a standard set of information was collected from all participants on admission. The treatment program, level of counselor training, and the observance of clinic procedures remained constant. Information was extracted from the complete set of 724 clinical charts and a comprehensive set of data, including demographic information, current and lifetime drug use, reasons for seeking treatment, family history of substance use, psychiatric history and existing psychological problems, self-reported health status and medical history, and legal status, was collected. There were also two standardized measures administered at admission which were derived to reflect self-reported problems related to stimulant use. For the purpose of this project, treatment progress was determined by using urine toxicology results collected randomly during treatment, by extracting information from detailed notes that indicated amount, type and frequency of clinical contact, and by compiling staff ratings of patient functioning at the time of discharge.

The Treatment Program. Treatment was based on the outpatient Matrix Model program,[7,8] which is designed to integrate several disparate interventions into a comprehensive, structured approach. Elements of the treatment included individual therapy, relapse prevention and family education groups, urine testing, and 12-step program involvement. Although there is a formal structure to the program, contents of the treatment materials are individualized to meet the needs of each specific client. The Matrix Model uses key cognitive-behavioral principles as the foundation of its program, with specific goals to: (1) stop drug use; (2) learn issues critical to addiction and relapse; (3) receive education for family members affected by addiction and recovery; (4) become familiar with self-help programs; and (5) receive weekly monitoring by urine toxicology and breath alcohol testing. Treatment materials for the Matrix program are manualized to aid in treatment standardization,[9] and this model is described more fully elsewhere.[7,8]

The recommended treatment duration for all treatment participants was 26 weeks from 1987-1990 and 16 weeks from 1991 to the present. Therefore, although the planned treatment stay shifted during the course of the study, it was changed for cocaine and methamphetamine users at the same time and did not affect comparison of the two groups.

RESULTS

Demographics. The demographics of those admitted to the clinic look similar to the county census: San Bernardino county population, where the clinic is located, is 73.1% Caucasian, 8.1% African-American, and 26.3% Hispanic.[10] However, there are significant demographic differences evident between methamphetamine and cocaine users (see Table 1). Specifically, a disproportionate number of the methamphetamine users were Caucasian (80.5%) while most of the cocaine users were non-Caucasian (52%). More than one-third of the cocaine users were African Americans (34.2%) compared to a small fraction of the methamphetamine users (1.9%). Overall, more male addicts using all substances sought treatment, but significantly more female methamphetamine users sought treatment than female cocaine users.

At admission, methamphetamine users were younger (M_{meth} =

TABLE 1. Demographic Information for Methamphetamine and Cocaine Users

		MA Users (n = 500)	Cocaine Users (n = 224)	Statistic and Significance
Gender†	Male	60.0%	68.8%	$X^2(1) = 5.1, p < .05$
	Female	40.0%	31.2%	
Ethnicity†	Caucasian	80.5%	48.0%	$X^2(2) = 151.0, p < .0001$
	Hispanic	16.7%	15.8%	
	African-American	1.9%	34.2%	
Marital Status†	Never Married	48.9%	36.1%	$X^2(2) = 15.9, p < .01$
	Married	25.8%	37.5%	
	Previously Married	25.3%	26.4%	
Employment†	Work Full Time	27.5%	31.2%	$X^2(2) = 9.7, p < .05$
	Work Part Time	10.8%	17.6%	
	Not Working	61.6%	50.9%	

†Numbers presented are percentages.

29.0 ± 6.5 years; $M_{cocaine}$ = 31.6 ± 6.7 years; $t_{(723)} = -4.9$ $p < .001$), and by several measures they were more disaffected than the cocaine users. This is apparent in the significantly lower level of education (M_{meth} = 11.8 ± 1.6; $M_{cocaine}$ = 12.4 ± 1.9), the lower rates of employment, and the lower rates of being in a stable relationship, compared to cocaine users (see Table 1).

Substance Use. Methamphetamine users started using stimulants at a younger age than did cocaine users (M_{meth} = 21.4 ± 6.7 years; $M_{cocaine}$ = 23.7 ± 7.2 years), and the pattern of use looks quite different (see Table 2). Cocaine users tend to binge, whereas nearly one half of the methamphetamine users use daily. It is interesting to note that cocaine users are significantly more likely to report that they are addicted to the drug and they are more likely to have received prior drug treatment.

TABLE 2. Primary Drug Use for Methamphetamine and Cocaine Users

		MA Users (n = 500)	Cocaine Users (n = 224)	Statistic and Significance
Age at First Use‡		21.4 (6.7)	23.7 (7.2)	$t_{(715)} = -4.2$, p < .001
Months of Heavy Use, Prior to Admission‡		41.2 (45.2)	39.7 (41.5)	n.s.
Route of Use†	Oral	1.2%	0.0%	$X^2(4) = 168$, p < .001
	Intranasal	55.4%	22.2%	
	Smoking	7.2%	48.0%	
	Multiple Non-IV Routes	22.6%	16.7%	
	Any IV Use	13.5%	13.1%	
Frequency of Use, Prior to Admission†	Less than once/week	16.6%	32.8%	$X^2(3) = 45.3$, p < .001
	1-2 times/week	21.3%	29.9%	
	3-6 times/week	14.5%	15.2%	
	Daily	47.7%	22.0%	
Feel Addicted†		82.1%	89.6%	$X^2(1) = 6.2$, p < .01
Had Prior Treatment†		24.6%	44.7%	$X^2(1) = 28.4$, p < .001

†Numbers presented are percentages.
‡Numbers presented are means and (standard deviations).

The two groups of stimulant addicts look quite different in their use of other substances. Not surprisingly, a substantial number of the cocaine users report frequent alcohol use, and this proportion is significantly higher than what is reported by the methamphetamine users (see Table 3). In contrast to this, methamphetamine users report more involvement in the past year with all other major classes of drugs than the cocaine users.

Response to Treatment. The results regarding the treatment experience of methamphetamine and cocaine users are presented in Table 4. As can be seen from these data, there is virtually no difference in the amount or type of treatment received. The two groups were retained in treatment for the same duration, and the survival curves for the two groups (see Figure 1) are nearly identical. Methamphetamine and cocaine users participated similarly in the program, with no significant differences in the number or frequency of "breaks" or interruptions in the course of treatment. In addition, treatment outcome, as measured by urine toxicology results, does not vary significantly between methamphetamine and cocaine users (see Table 4).

TABLE 3. Other Drug and Alcohol Use for Methamphetamine and Cocaine Users

		MA Users (n = 500)	Cocaine Users (n = 224)	Statistic and Significance
Alcohol Use†	More than Once Weekly	22.5%	31.1%	$X^2(2) = 21.6, p < .001$
	Weekly or monthly	43.7%	48.8%	
	Never use	33.8%	20.1%	
Alcohol†	Use w/ Primary Drug	34.3%	46.9%	$X^2(1) = 9.9, p < .01$
	Need Alcohol Treatment	12.6%	24.6%	$X^2(1) = 14.9, p < .001$
Other Drug Use, in Past Year†	Cocaine	10.8%	100.0%	$X^2(2) = 520, p < .001$
	Methamphetamine	100.0%	17.9%	$X^2(2) = 550, p < .001$
	Marijuana	56.2%	42.4%	$X^2(2) = 11.8, p < .001$
	Hallucinogens/PCP	6.4%	0.0%	$X^2(2) = 15.0, p < .001$
	Opiates	4.6%	6.2%	n.s.
	Barbiturates	2.8%	2.2%	n.s.

†Numbers presented are percentages.
‡Numbers presented are means and (standard deviations).

TABLE 4. Treatment Experience for Methamphetamine and Cocaine Users

		MA Users (n = 500)	Cocaine Users (n = 224)	Statistic and Significance
Treatment Received, In Number of Hours‡	Individual Sessions	13.3 (13.6)	16.3 (15.3)	$t_{(721)} = -2.6, p < .01$
	Early Recovery Group	3.4 (4.4)	3.7 (3.3)	n.s.
	Relapse Prevention Group	23.7 (29.0)	21.0 (26.8)	n.s.
	Family Education Group	11.6 (14.0)	12.2 (12.8)	n.s.
	Social Support Group	4.4 (14.9)	4.3 (18.2)	n.s.
Number of Breaks in Treatment‡		0.4 (1.1)	0.5 (1.3)	n.s.
Total of Treatment Hours Received‡		52.9 (51.4)	54.5 (49.3)	n.s.
Weeks in Treatment‡		17.1 (22.3)	18.0 (21.3)	n.s.
Urine Samples Collected‡		8.3 (8.0)	8.1 (7.6)	n.s.
Percentage of Samples Positive (Dirty) for Primary Drug†		19.3%	13.3%	n.s.

†Numbers presented are percentages.
‡Numbers presented are means and (standard deviations).

DISCUSSION

Much of the treatment experience with methamphetamine abusers dates back some twenty-five years and primarily deals with the acute medical complications seen with intoxication or withdrawal. The emphasis on the treatment of dependence and prevention of relapse for methamphetamine abuse/dependence has been a more recent endeavor. Most of the current strategies for treating methamphetamine abuse and dependence are borrowed from experiences with treating cocaine addicts. Recent indications of the spread of methamphetamine abuse has converted a regional issue into a problem calling for a national response.

This sense of urgency may result in precipitous responses by the treatment and research community unless careful consideration is

FIGURE 1

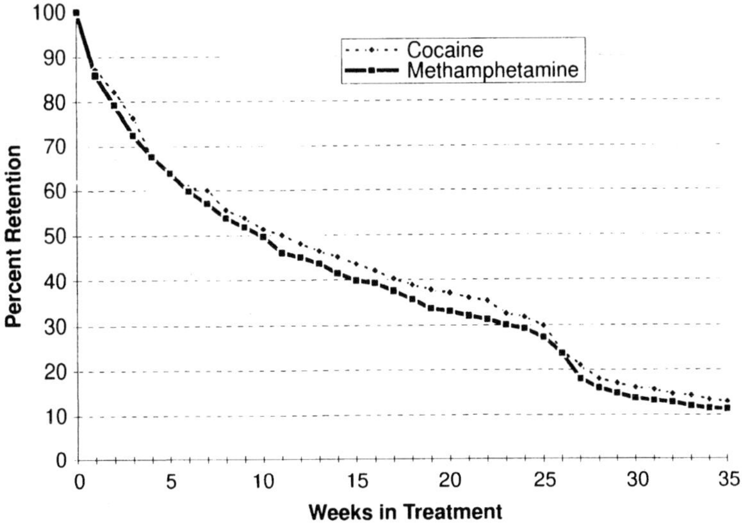

given to the lessons learned from earlier experience with cocaine, especially in the area of integrated treatment approaches. The temptation to view cocaine and methamphetamine as similar stimulants will likely lead to the reevaluation of many of the same compounds used in earlier trials although some fundamental differences in the mechanism of action between cocaine and methamphetamine have been identified.[11,12,13] At the clinical level, the testing of a pharmacotherapeutic strategy is likely to involve some psychosocial support which alone could be expected to contribute a certain amount of treatment response. It is necessary to understand the degree to which treatment response is attributable to psychosocial interventions in order to reasonably assess the success or failure of the added pharmacotherapy. Such information has been virtually nonexistent in the recent literature. The present findings do suggest that there is a measurable degree of response of methamphetamine abusers to psychosocial intervention, and that the general treatment experience, as reflected by the attendance of therapeutic sessions, breaks in treatment participation, and total treatment received, does not differ significantly between methamphetamine and cocaine users. Such findings provide a benchmark against which a treatment effect of added pharmacotherapy can be measured and lend some confidence to the notion that in similar settings pharmacotherapeutic interventions can have either an additive or synergistic effect with psychosocial treatments.

REFERENCES

1. Heischober B, Miller M. Methamphetamine abuse in California. NIDA Research Monograph 1991;115:60-71.

2. Substance Abuse and Mental Health Services Administration (1995b). Drug Abuse Warning Network, October, 1995.

3. Substance Abuse and Mental Health Services Administration (1995a). National Household Survey on Drug Abuse: Population Estimates, 1994.

4. Frosch D, Shoptaw S, Huber A, Rawson R, Ling W. Sexual HIV risk among gay and bisexual male methamphetamine abusers. J Subst Abuse Treat. 1996; 13(4):1-4.

5. Ling W, Shoptaw S. Integration of research in pharmacotherapy for addictive disease. Where are we? Where are we going? J Addict Dis. 1997;16(4): 83-102.

6. Cunningham JK, Thielemier MA. Trends and regional variations in amphetamine-related emergency admissions: California, 1984-1993. CA: Public Statistics Institute, 1995.

7. Rawson R, Obert JL, McCann MJ, Ling W. Psychological approaches for the treatment of cocaine dependence–a neurobehavioral approach. J Addict Dis. 1991;11(2):97-120.

8. Shoptaw S, Rawson RA, McCann MJ, Obert JL. The Matrix model of outpatient stimulant abuse treatment: evidence of efficacy. J Addict Dis. 1994;13(4): 129-141.

9. Rawson R, Obert J, McCann M, Smith D, Scheffey EH. The Neurobehavioral Treatment Manual, Matrix: Los Angeles, CA, 1989.

10. US Census Bureau (1990). 1990 Census of San Bernardino County, California.

11. Ritz MC, Kuhar MJ. Relationship between self-administration of amphetamine and monamine receptors in brain: comparison with cocaine. J Pharmacol Exp Ther. 1989;248(2):1010-1017.

12. Loh EA, Roberts DS. Break-points on a progressive ratio schedule reinforced by intravenous cocaine increase following depletion of forebrain serotonin. Psychopharmacology 1990;101:262-266.

13. Roberts DS. Self-administration of stimulants and serotonergic systems. NIDA Research Monograph 1992;199:136-140.

The Integration of Pharmacotherapy and Nonpharmacotherapy

Norman S. Miller, MD
David E. Smith, MD

THE INTEGRATION OF PHARMACOTHERAPY AND PSYCHOSOCIAL THERAPIES IN THE TREATMENT OF ADDICTIVE DISEASE

While pharmacotherapies have been employed in the treatment of drug and alcohol addiction, their use has been largely limited to the treatment of detoxification (withdrawal states). The recent interest to prevent relapse (addiction states) is new and in the early stages of development. Clinical attitudes of physicians toward pharmacological treatments and bias against traditional treatment methods have motivated research in pharmacotherapies for addictive disorders.[1]

Studies on disulfiram and naltrexone suggest that medications can be used to enhance compliance with nonpharmacological or traditional psychosocial forms of addictions treatment. The devel-

---

Norman S. Miller is affiliated with the Department of Psychiatry, The University of Illinois at Chicago, Chicago, IL. David E. Smith is affiliated with the Haight Ashbury Free Clinics, San Francisco, CA.

Address correspondence to: Norman S. Miller, MD, The University of Illinois at Chicago, Department of Psychiatry (M/C 913), 912 South Wood Street, Chicago, IL 60612-7327.

[Haworth co-indexing entry note]: "The Integration of Pharmacotherapy and Nonpharmacotherapy." Miller, Norman S., and David E. Smith. Co-published simultaneously in *Journal of Addictive Diseases* (The Haworth Medical Press, an imprint of The Haworth Press, Inc.) Vol. 16, No. 4, 1997, pp. 51-64; and: *The Integration of Pharmacological and Nonpharmacological Treatments in Drug/Alcohol Addictions* (ed: Norman S. Miller, and Barry Stimmel) The Haworth Medical Press, an imprint of The Haworth Press, Inc., 1997, pp. 51-64. Single or multiple copies of this article are available for a fee from The Haworth Document Delivery Service [1-800-342-9678, 9:00 a.m. - 5:00 p.m. (EST). E-mail address: getinfo@haworth.com].

opment of medications aimed to improve engagement and retention, and ultimately compliance with addictions treatment are being increasingly considered and studied.[2-4]

THE INDEPENDENT STATUS FOR ADDICTIVE DISORDERS IN MEDICATION DEVELOPMENT: THE DISEASE STATE

Progressive changes in the Diagnostic and Statistical Manuals have formed a basis for the acceptance of substance-related disorders as independent diseases. The movement away from underlying causes for drug and alcohol use is evident from a comparison of *DSM-I* where addictive disorders were considered as a personality disorder to the current *DSM-IV* where the diagnosis of substance-related disorders takes predominance over other psychiatric disorders. Exclusionary criteria contained in most psychiatric disorders require the effects of substance-related disorders be excluded before another psychiatric diagnosis can be made independently.[5]

The interest in pharmacotherapies in the treatment of addictive disorders reinforces the credibility of their disease state. The assumption for the development of medications specially for addictive diseases is an independent status with characteristic etiology, course, and prognosis. In general, medications are used for diseases in order to alter course. A disease is usually regarded as a state where the victim is helpless, passive, and not at fault, and treatment with medication is a relatively passive process. However, the notion of personal responsibility in initiating treatment and sustaining recovery in addictive illness is fundamental to the therapeutic response in many medical illnesses. While medications work passively, the patient must be actively compliant with taking them to achieve success.[1,6]

The notion that alcohol and drug use is conditional on psychological states or psychiatric illness has not been productive in the development of pharmacotherapies or therapies in general for addictive diseases. The self-medication hypothesis in drug and alcohol use has not been proven in any objective way. Studies actually show the lack of medication benefit by alcohol and drug use, and a worsening of rationalized symptoms in addictive alcohol and drug use. The notion of self-medication is counterproductive to the integration of medications with other forms of addiction treatments. Directing medications at perceived "underlying causes" of addictive disease will result in treating conditions unrelated to drug and alcohol use and addiction.[7,8]

A rational approach to addictive disease requires an understanding of the etiological nature or vulnerability to the development of compulsive drug use, and the brain mechanisms involved in the loss of control evident in addictive drug use. Specific areas in the limbic system of the brain appear responsible for drug and alcohol use, namely, the mesolimbic pathway which extends from the ventral tegmental area (VTA) to the nucleus accumbens (NA).[9]

The spirit of medication development and the integration of pharmacotherapies with traditional methods of addiction treatment, which are largely nonpharmacological, will be in the patient's benefit. We have effective treatments for drug and alcohol addiction in the form of cognitive behavioral therapies and the participation in 12-step groups in long-term recovery. A polar approach to the treatment of addictive disorders of either pharmacological or nonpharmacological will not be productive for optimal patient care. The challenges to the integration of these seemingly divergent approaches are great. However, the promise of improved outcome for our patients with addictive disease is worth the effort and attendant changes.[10-12]

VULNERABILITY FOR ADDICTIVE DISEASES

Environmental factors have always played a role in the development and propagation of addictive diseases. A simple equation of exposure (environmental) plus vulnerability (genetic) equals addiction can be used to illustrate fundamental concepts in the origin of addictive disease. A widely believed notion is that supply of alcohol and other drugs is fundamental to its use, particularly in vulnerable individuals. Moreover, other psychosocial factors play important roles in the onset and propagation of drug use and addiction; peer influence and involvement with drugs can predict who will develop problematic use of alcohol and drugs and eventual complications from addictive alcohol and drug use.[13]

Genetic predisposition is a predictor of who possesses the vulnerability to drug and alcohol addiction. Familial, twin, adoption, and high risk studies have supported a substantial role for genetic factors in predicting the onset of alcoholism and drug addiction. The single best predictor of who will develop addictive disease is a history of such addictive disease in family members (blood relatives). Alcoholism and drug addiction run strongly in families; greater than 50% of alcoholics and drug addicts will have at least one family member with alcoholism or drug addiction, and likely to have more than one family member affected. Monozygotic twins are more concordant for alcohol and drug addiction than dizygotic twins. Adoptees with a biological parent with alcohol or drug addiction are more likely to develop addictive disease than adoptees without such a genetic background. Sons and daughters of alcoholics were more likely to show behavioral and biological correlates of alcoholism than those without such a genetic background.[14]

NEUROCHEMISTRY

Perhaps the most rational basis for medication development is identification of neurochemical pathways underlying addictive use of drugs and alcohol. The mesolimbic pathway in subcortical brain regions has been shown to be important in the self-administration of alcohol and drugs in animals, and probably underlies compulsive use of alcohol and drugs in humans. The mesolimbic pathway is important in the reinforcement of eating and sexual behaviors, and its function suggests that addictive use of alcohol and drugs is related to instinctual drive states such as hunger and sex that are stereotypic, repetitive, and relentless in their expression.[9]

The mesolimbic pathway extends from the ventral tegmentum (VT) in the midbrain to the nucleus accumbens (NA) in the limbic forebrain. Several neurotransmitters subserve these structures; principally dopamine (DA) neurons in the VT that extend to the NA, and opiate neurons that synapse on DA neurons. Serotonin (5-HT) and GABA neurons synapse with other neurons to modulate mesolimbic activity. Other peptides and neurotransmitters synapse at various sites to participate in a cascade of neurotransmission for addictive drug use. Alcohol, cocaine, cannabis, nicotine, and opiates stimulate these neurotransmitters and peptides to activate the complex circuitry in addictive disease. Many medications tried thus far have been targeted at these neurotransmitters and peptides and limbic areas of the brain.[9,15]

The limbic system also subserves mood states, e.g., anxiety and depression. Medications for addictive illness often have side effects on mood and other appetites. A balance to suppress appetitive drives and mood states will be a challenge to medication development.[9,15]

CLINICAL INDICATIONS AND SPECIFIC BRAIN TARGETS FOR CURRENT MEDICATIONS

Medications used in addictive disease can be classified according to clinical uses and brain actions. Clinical uses generally include the treatment of acute withdrawal (detoxification) and relapse prevention (addiction). Understanding their mechanisms of actions is part of a rational approach to the development of medications specific to addictive disease.[16-18]

Cross Tolerance and Dependence. Benzodiazepines are effective in detoxification from alcohol. They act by suppressing withdrawal from alcohol due to the pharmacological cross tolerance and dependence between alcohol and benzodiazepines. Benzodiazepines and alcohol appear to influence GABA transmission, the former by acting on specific receptor sites, and the latter by acting on neuronal membranes in the brain.[16-18]

Antagonists. Disulfiram acts by competitively inhibiting acetaldehyde dehydrogenase, and promoting an accumulation of noxious metabolite acetaldehyde when alcohol is ingested. Naltrexone may act by competitively inhibiting opiate receptors on the dopamine neurons in the mesolimbic pathway. Disulfiram and naltrexone have been shown effective as adjuncts in conjunction with psychosocial forms of treatment. Other medications with less impressive findings are antidepressants; tricyclic antidepressants and selective serotonin reuptake inhibition antidepressants act by competitively inhibiting reuptake at postsynaptic sites.[16-18]

Antiepileptic. Carbamazepine and valproic acid have been studied in alcohol and drug withdrawal. The putative mechanism of action is suppression of the firing of a repetitive focus, in the limbic area. Withdrawal is characterized by sympathetic stimulation, and excitable levels of arousal in the brain, particularly, in subcortical brain regions.[19]

Agonists. Clonidine acts at presynaptic norepinephrine sites in the locus ceruleus to suppress the excessive release of norepinephrine during opiate and alcohol withdrawal. The α-2 receptors are also suppressed by release of norepinephrine in a feedback mechanism under normal conditions. Methadone acts on opiate receptors in the locus ceruleus and VTA to replace effects of other opiates, namely heroin, to reduce its use.[19]

TRADITIONAL ADDICTIONS TREATMENT (NONPHARMACOLOGICAL OR PSYCHOSOCIAL)

The predominant form of addictions treatment employs the abstinence-based methods. The abstinence based methods include acceptance of drug and alcohol addictions as an independent disease that has an identifiable and predictable course and prognosis, and responds to specific addictions treatment approaches. The specific treatment methods include cognitive behavior therapies in group and individual settings. Abstinence is the goal, and reinforced in expectations and contracts around program participation and completion. Most abstinence-based programs utilize 12-step recovery programs, and make regular referrals to Alcoholics Anonymous and Narcotics Anonymous.[12]

A national survey found the abstinence-based methods to be used by over 95% of the treatment centers reviewed. The disease concept was employed, and the programs were based on the "12-step program" of Alcoholics Anonymous. Abstinence was the only accepted goal for any patient ultimately in recovery.[20]

Two controlled studies have found the abstinence-based method of treatment effective. In one study, a randomized clinical trial showed the "Hazelden" type of abstinence-based treatment to be more effective than traditional forms of treatment. One hundred forty-one employed alcoholics were randomly assigned to either the Hazelden program (N = 74) or the traditional type treatment (N = 67). The Hazelden method was significantly more involving and supportive, encouraging spontaneity and oriented to personal problems. The dropout rate was 7.9% for the Hazelden and 25.9% for the traditional, one year abstinence was greater for the former than latter type of treatment.[10]

In the other controlled study, a random assignment of 227 employees who were diagnosed as alcoholics and cocaine addicts was made to inpatient, outpatient, or choice (inpatient, outpatient or referral to AA). On seven measures of drinking and drug use, the inpatient group showed significantly superior abstinence and overall treatment outcome, followed by the choice group, and then the AA group. While direct referral to the AA group was the least effective, ultimately both the inpatient and outpatient groups were referred to AA.[11]

In evaluation studies of largely employed alcoholics and drug addicts, a sample of 8,087 inpatients and 1,663 outpatients showed impressive treatment outcome at one year. The contact rate for one year postdischarge was 70%. The results showed an overall abstinence rate of 55% regardless of postdischarge disposition. The abstinence rates improved progressively to 70-80% for those who attended continuing care and/or AA out to one year.[21] (See Table.)

In another study of largely unemployed alcoholics and drug addicts, a sample of 133 inpatients was followed for six months. The contact rate was 57%. An abstinence rate of 57% was achieved for six months if the patients attended AA and the aftercare clinic. Thirty percent were attending the aftercare clinic at 6 months.[22]

Other forms of treatment than abstinence-based have been stud-

TABLE

One-Year Abstinence by Continuum of Care and Self-Help Support

Variable		Inpatients (n = 6508)		Outpatients (n = 1572)	
		% Attending	% Abstinent	% Attending	% Abstinent
Months of continuing care attended in year:					
	0	42	53	34	48
	1-5	32	55	33	61
	6-11	19	71	18	68
	12	8	88	14	89
AA attendance:	Non-attender	54	47	43	49
	Regular attender	46	74	57	80

Table is from Miller NS, Hoffmann NG. Addictions treatment outcomes. Alcohol Treat Q. 1995; 12(2):41-55.

ied in controlled trials, often recognized by terms such as relapse prevention, social skills training, and motivational enhancement. No large-scale evaluation studies of these methods have been performed. Included in these studies is a large variance in methods, numbers of subjects (often small), inclusions of unstandardized diagnoses, e.g., alcohol problems, and short follow-up, e.g., weeks to a few months. Patient selection bias made randomization often questionable. Also, the relevance to the contemporary alcoholic is limited because patients with alcohol diagnoses and/or drug problems or diagnoses were often excluded. Most of these methods are rarely used clinically and cannot be recommended as the standard of care.[12,23-36]

MEDICATION TRIALS

The medications best studied have been methadone, disulfiram, and recently naltrexone. In general, the studies show the best results were obtained when medications are combined with psychosocial forms of treatments. Treatment outcome is greatly enhanced in methadone maintenance programs if behavioral and social programs are given in addition to methadone. Disulfiram was found to be useful as an adjunct to other psychosocial forms of treatment, particularly in those patients who were motivated for abstinence from alcohol. Naltrexone in two controlled studies was shown to be more effective than placebo at three months postdischarge. Naltrexone and placebo were administered in conjunction with psychosocial forms of treatment although these were experimental and not the standard forms of abstinence-based treatments generally employed in clinical practice.[3,4]

While many controlled and uncontrolled studies have examined pharmacological forms of treatment for cocaine addiction, no medications can be recommended for clinical practice at this time. Early, promising studies were not replicated in later studies.[16-18]

NATURAL HISTORY OF RELAPSE AND TREATMENT RESPONSE

We know from studies that drug and alcohol addictions are chronic, relapsing disorders, particularly in the untreated state. According to the Epidemiological Catchment Area Studies (ECA), 50% of alcoholics and drug addicts were in active use of alcohol and drugs. In longitudinal studies, the likelihood of abstaining from alcohol was 20% without treatment. In studies of treatment populations, the greatest number of relapses occurred within the first month (50%), and within six months (80%). These rates appeared generalizable to many forms of treatment and drug types (alcohol, heroin, cocaine), and reflect intrinsic characteristics of the addictive illness.[37]

We know we can offset these relapse rates with treatment interventions and longer-term recovery. The treatment process can be considered as engagement, retention, referral, and recovery. Most of our studies involve outcome in retention and recovery. In the studies of naltrexone, the number and severity of relapses were reduced. In evaluation studies, the longer the patient is retained in continuing care and AA, the greater the abstinence rates and improved treatment outcome. However, the compliance rates for naltrexone was 60% at three months and 20% at one year for continuing care for abstinence and 45% for attendance at AA.[38]

The studies suggest that a potential role for medications is in combination with psychosocial forms of treatment to enhance engagement and retention with treatment and eventual long-term recovery rates. For instance, if we can increase compliance with continuing care and AA, e.g., increased numbers retained from 20% and 45%, the treatment effect can be expected to result in greater abstinence and improved treatment outcome.[12] The naltrexone studies suggest that the medication benefit can extend to reducing relapse and severity of relapses.

We know from many studies of detoxification that the use of medications can enhance engagement and retention during the early, acute withdrawal states, e.g., the first few days of abstinence. The use of medications beyond acute detoxification such as naltrexone could enhance compliance with standard forms of treatments, e.g., abstinence-based methods.

CHARACTERISTICS OF MEDICATIONS IN ADDICTIVE DISORDERS

The ideal medication is one that has efficacy without toxicity. Few if any medications in medicine have these characteristics.

Nonetheless it is important to keep in mind certain relative contraindications in alcoholics and drug addicts regarding their vulnerability to medications. First, no harmful drug interactions between medications and drugs of addiction, e.g., overdose potential. Second, no potential for the development of addiction or pharmacological dependence that can neutralize the positive benefits of the medications. Third, side effects that do not impede recovery such as suppression of emotions, impairment of cognition and blunting of energy and motivational states in recovery. Alcoholics and drug addicts possess greater vulnerability to the adverse effects and development of alcohol and drug addiction to wide range of medications than those who do not possess a history of addiction.

POSSIBLE INDICATIONS FOR CURRENT USE OF MEDICATIONS

The indications for adjunctive medications are relatively uncharted beyond their use in detoxification. Three major areas that can be targeted are settings, severity and comorbidity. In general, medications can be used in outpatient settings to improve compliance and reduce relapse to alcohol and drugs. Studies tend to support the notion that patients with greater severity are selected for inpatient settings, and that otherwise the treatment outcomes are similar for inpatient and outpatient settings. Moreover, studies tend to show that patients with severe addiction severity experience greater relapse rates and poorer treatment outcome no matter what the setting. Also, those with psychiatric comorbidity, particularly, the chronic mentally ill appear to have fewer opportunities for traditional forms of addictions treatment.

The use of medications in these patient populations appears warranted, particularly, those such as naltrexone and disulfiram, in conjunction with other forms of treatment. Interestingly, while much has been written about the importance of addiction and psychiatric severity in influencing treatment outcome, little has been documented in actual studies. Most available studies actually show that severity from multiple causes, medical, addiction and psychiatric, actually prompts patients to seek treatment in greater numbers than those without severity.

In a study of depressed alcoholics and cocaine addicts, compliance with treatment programs and attendance at self-help groups was greater in those with a history of major depression. No difference was found in abstinence rates and treatment outcome as measured by medical, psychiatric, and legal consequences. Other studies show that depression is not necessarily a predictor of poorer treatment outcome.

The few available studies on the addicted chronically mentally ill suggest that they can respond to addictions treatment and utilize self-help groups similarly to those who are addicted without psychiatric comorbidity. Most of these patients are on medications for their mental illness.

FUNDAMENTAL CONCEPTS ABOUT MEDICATIONS

The notion of medications for addiction appears in conflict with fundamental beliefs regarding drugs held by the "recovering community." The first is that a "drug solution" has not worked for addicts, and in fact has increased the morbidity and mortality in their lives. The addict has a fundamental defect in controlling drug use of potentially any kind, and drugs including medications can induce subtle alterations in cognition, feelings and beliefs regarding recovery. The basis for recovery for many in self-help groups is away from a reliance on drugs to solve problems and alter beliefs and feelings, and towards cognitive-behavioral changes that are inner directed and personal responsibility towards abstinence and maturation.

The use of medications must somehow reconcile reliance on self to change with reliance on a medication to change self. The two appear contradictory but not necessarily irreconcilable. However, a fundamental understanding of recovery from addictive illness and the limitations of medications are necessary to begin integrating the two seemingly dichotomous approaches.

For alcoholics and drug addicts, the spiritual changes that they experience are of an educational variety. William James describes spiritual experiences that develop slowly over a period of time, where quite often the friends of the alcoholic are aware of differences long before him or her. The addict eventually experiences a profound alteration in reactions to life; that such a change could hardly have been brought about by the individual alone.

REFERENCES

1. Miller NS, Gold MS. The psychiatrist's role in integrating pharmacologic and nonpharmacologic treatments for addictive disorders. Psychiatr Ann. 1992; 22:436-40.

2. Fuller RK, Branchey L, Brightwell DR, Derman RM, Emrick CD, Iber FL, James KE, Lacoursiere RB, Lee KK, Lowenstam I, Maany I, Neiderhiser D, Nocks JJ, Shaw S. Disulfiram treatment of alcoholism: a Veterans Administration cooperative study. JAMA. 1986; 256:1449-55.

3. Volpicelli JR, Alterman AI, Hayashida M, O'Brien CP. Naltrexone in the treatment of alcohol dependence. Arch Gen Psychiatry. 1992; 49:876-80.

4. O'Malley SS, Jaffee AJ, Chang S, Schottenfield RS, Meyer RE, Rounsaville B. Naltrexone and coping skills therapy for alcohol dependence: a controlled study. Arch Gen Psychiatry. 1992; 49:881-7.

5. Diagnostic and statistical manual. Fourth edition. American Psychiatric Association. Washington, DC, 1995.

6. Miller NS, Chappel JN. The history of the disease concept. Psychiatr Ann. 1991; 21(1):1-8.

7. Tamerin JS, Mendelson JH. The psychodynamics of chronic inebriation: observations of alcoholics during the process of drinking in an experimental group setting. Am J Psychiatry. 1969; 125:886-99.

8. Miller NS, Mahler JC, Belkin BM, Gold MS. Psychiatric diagnosis in alcohol and drug dependence. Ann Clin Psychiatry. 1991; 3:79-89.

9. Miller NS, Gold MS. A neurochemical basis for alcohol and other drug addiction. J Psychoactive Drugs. 1993; 25(2):121-8.

10. Keso L, Salaspuro M. Inpatient treatment of employed alcoholics: a randomized clinical trial on Hazelden-type and traditional treatment. Alcohol Clin Exp Res. 1990; 14:584-9.

11. Walsh EC, Hingson RW, Merrigan DM, et al. A randomized trial of treatment options for alcohol abusing workers. N Engl J Med. 1991; 325:775-82.

12. Miller NS. Treatment of the addictions: Applications of outcome research for clinical management. New York: Haworth Press, 1995.

13. Dupré D, Miller NS, Gold MS. Initiation and progression of alcohol, marijuana and cocaine use among adolescent abusers. Am J Addict. 1995; 4(1):43-8.

14. Miller NS. Generalized vulnerability to drug and alcohol addiction. In: Miller NS, ed. The principles and practices of addictions in psychiatry. Philadelphia: W.B. Saunders, in press.

15. Miller NS, Gold MS. Abuse, addiction, tolerance and dependence to benzodiazepines: in medical and nonmedical populations. Am J Alcohol Drug Abuse. 1991; 17:27-39.

16. Liskow BI, Goodwin DW. Pharmacological treatment of alcohol intoxication, withdrawal and dependence: a critical review. J Stud Alcohol. 1987; 8:356-70.

17. Litten RZ, Allen JP. Pharmacotherapies for alcoholism: promising agents and clinical issues. Alcohol Clin Exp Res. 1991; 15(4):620-33.

18. Gorelick DA. Overview of pharmacological treatment approaches for alcohol and other drug addiction. Intoxication, withdrawal, and relapse prevention. Psychiatr Clin North Am. 1993; 16(1):141-56.

19. Miller NS, Gold MS. Pharmacological therapies for drug and alcohol addiction. New York: Marcel Dekker, Inc., 1995.

20. Roman P. Inpatient alcohol and drug treatment centers. Executive report. National Institute on Alcohol Abuse and Alcoholism, 1989.

21. Hoffmann NG, Miller NS. Treatment outcome for abstinence-based programs. Psychiatr Ann. 1992; 22:402-7.

22. Miller NS, Verinis S. Treatment outcome on impoverished alcoholics in an abstinence-based program. Int J Addict. 1995; 30(6):753-63.

23. Cannon DS, Baker TB, Wehl CK. Emetic and electric shock alcohol aversion therapy: Six- and twelve-month follow-up. J Consult Clin Psychol. 1981; 49:360-8.

24. Chaney EF, O'Leary MR, Marlatt GA. Skill training with alcoholics. J Consult Clin Psychol. 1978; 46:1092-1104.

25. Edwards G, Guthrie S. A comparison of inpatient and outpatient treatment of alcohol dependence. Lancet. 1966; 1:467-8.

26. Edwards G, Guthrie S. A controlled trial of inpatient and outpatient treatment of alcohol dependence. Lancet. 1967; 1:555-9.

27. Emerick CD. A review of psychologically oriented treatment of alcoholism. I. The use and interrelations of outcome criteria and drunken behavior following treatment. Q J Stud Alcohol. 1974; 35:523.

28. Emerick CD. A review of psychologically oriented treatment of alcoholism: II. Q J Stud Alcohol. 1975;36(1):88-103.

29. Ends EJ, Page CW. A study of three types of group psychotherapy with hospitalized inebriates. Q J Stud Alcohol. 1957;18:263-77.

30. Miller NS. Special problems of the alcohol and multiple-drug dependent: clinical interactions and detoxification. In: Frances RJ, Miller SI, eds. Clinical textbook of addictive disorders. New York: The Guilford Press, 1991:194-218.

31. Marlatt GA. A comparison of aversive conditioning procedures in the treatment of alcoholism. Paper presented at the annual meeting of the Western Psychological Association, Anaheim, CA, 1993: April.

32. McCance C, McCance PF. Alcoholism in North-East Scotland: its treatment and outcome. Br J Psychiatry. 1969; 115:189-98.

33. Ogborne AC, Wilmot R. Evaluation of an experimental counseling service for male Skid Row alcoholics. J Stud Alcohol. 1979; 40:129-32.

34. Pendery ML, Maltzman TM, West LJ. Controlled drinking by alcoholics? New findings and a re-evaluation of a major affirmative study. Science. 1982; 217:169-75.

35. Rosenberg SD. Relaxation training and a differential assessment of alcoholism. Unpublished doctoral dissertation, California School of Professional Psychology, San Diego, CA, 1979: University Microfilms No. 8004362.

36. Schaefer HH, Sobell MB, Mills KC. Some sobering data on the use of self-confrontation with alcoholics. Behav Ther. 1971; 2:28-39.

37. Miller NS, Gold MS. The role of the psychiatrist in treatment of relapse in addictive disorders. Psychiatr Ann. 1995; 25(11):673-8.

38. Chappel J. Long term recovery from alcoholism. In: Miller NS, ed. Psychiatric clinics of North America. Philadelphia: W.B. Saunders, Co., 1993:177-89.

Integration of Pharmacotherapies in the Existing Programs for the Treatment of Alcoholics: An International Perspective

Flavio Poldrugo, MD, PhD

SUMMARY. This review examines current therapies of alcoholism and addresses the difficulties encountered in evaluating the result of integrating pharmaco- and psychosocial treatment of alcoholics. A variety of treatment modalities and goals, and factors influencing admission of alcoholics, exist in different countries creating problems of comparability.

Recognition of alcoholism as a separate entity from associated psychiatric co-morbidity coupled with the introduction of specific pharmacotherapies represent a major advance in the treatment of alcoholism.

Combining psychosocial and pharmacological treatments appears to be the most effective approach in the treatment of alcoholics. In the future, rational therapy with appropriate choice of treatment strategies will decrease the necessity for hospital treatment of alcoholic patients. *[Article copies available for a fee from The Haworth Document Delivery Service: 1-800-342-9678. E-mail address: getinfo@haworth.com]*

Flavio Poldrugo is affiliated with the Department of Psychiatry, Alcohol and Related Addictions Research Group, University of Trieste, 34126 Trieste, Italy.

Address correspondence to: Flavio Poldrugo, MD, PhD, Alcohol and Related Addictions Research Group, Department of Psychiatry, School of Medicine, Via San Cilino 16, 34126 Trieste, Italy.

[Haworth co-indexing entry note]: "Integration of Pharmacotherapies in the Existing Programs for the Treatment of Alcoholics: An International Perspective." Poldrugo, Flavio. Co-published simultaneously in *Journal of Addictive Diseases* (The Haworth Medical Press, an imprint of The Haworth Press, Inc.) Vol. 16, No. 4, 1997, pp. 65-82; and: *The Integration of Pharmacological and Nonpharmacological Treatments in Drug/Alcohol Addictions* (ed: Norman S. Miller, and Barry Stimmel) The Haworth Medical Press, an imprint of The Haworth Press, Inc., 1997, pp. 65-82. Single or multiple copies of this article are available for a fee from The Haworth Document Delivery Service [1-800-342-9678, 9:00 a.m. - 5:00 p.m. (EST). E-mail address: getinfo@haworth.com].

INTRODUCTION

For many years, the medical management of alcoholism was based almost entirely on psychotherapeutic and psychosocial treatments, ranging from self-help groups to behavioral therapy. While these approaches still have a major part to play, recent studies have revealed exciting new possibilities in terms of potential pharmacological tools integrated in a general strategy of treatment of the alcoholic patient.

Many difficulties are encountered in general in drawing conclusions concerning the effects of alcoholism treatment. Some of these are related to the definition and measure of outcome, whereas others are concerned with factors such as measurement of an often fluctuating alcohol consumption level, the possible impact of spontaneous remission, the diverse heterogeneity and types of alcoholics within any particular study population, and the wide differences existing in treatment modalities, goals, and settings.

Although most clinical researchers consider the patient group under investigation as a representative sample of the population in which the study is being conducted, clinical investigators generally tend to select more "vulnerable" patients; those showing marked physical and mental impairments.

Cultural and Related Aspects

Patterns of Drinking

The culture and the pattern of drinking vary in different countries. Thus, countries characterized by "binge drinking" (e.g., Finland, Sweden and Canada) have more treatment facilities, since it has been demonstrated that the number of treatment programs reflects the extent of behavioral consequences of drinking and the proportion of beverages consumed as spirits[1] (Table 1). By contrast, countries where continuous wine consumption is integrated in dietary habits (like Italy and France), and whose global alcohol consumption is 2-3 times greater, have fewer treatment facilities. In the Mediterranean countries, spontaneous remission is rare, and alcoholics are treated in medical wards because of prominent physical disturbances (e.g., liver cirrhosis, G.I. tract diseases, pancreatitis, etc.).[2]

TABLE 1. Density of Alcoholism Treatment, Alcohol Consumption, and Liver Cirrhosis Mortality

Treatment extent rank	Alcohol consumption/ liters (1980)	Share of spirits (1980)	Death due to cirrhosis (1987)	
			Male	Female
1. Finland	6.3	44%	11.8	5.5
2. Sweden	5.4	44%	9.5	5.1
3. Switzerland	11.5	20%	16.9	6.4
4. New Zealand	8.6	22%	4.4	2.5
5. Canada	8.8	38%	11.2	5.7
6. U.S.A.	10.5	35%	14.4	7.3
7. U.K.	7.3	23%	6.4	5.2
8. Austria	11.0	15%	38.3	14.6
9. Italy	13.0	15%	42.0	19.7
10. France	16.3	21%	29.2	11.5

Health Policies and Legislation

Existing health policies are also a very important factor. In Europe, to give an example, most of the programs for alcoholics are provided to all citizens directly by the public services. In the U.S.A., instead, the health system operates through the private and public markets and alcoholics are inevitably selected for treatment on the basis of their economic resources (and type of insurance coverage).[3] Also the philosophy underlying public intervention for alcohol and drug addiction varies among different countries, thus directing different types of alcoholics to different treatment facilities. For example, in Europe, legislations may be limited to either alcohol problems (e.g., Hungary), or drug problems (e.g., Italy); or both either separately (e.g., Sweden) or combined (e.g., Finland). Alternatively, addiction may be covered by mental health acts (e.g., U.K.).[4] Some countries consider also compulsory treatment, but the grounds for intervention vary from the need of caring for the alcoholic's family (e.g., Switzerland), to the need of curing alcohol-related ailments (e.g., with special reference to mental health in the U.K.), or to control public order (e.g., Finland) and social conformity (e.g., legislation in former Soviet Union).[5]

NON-PHARMACOLOGICAL INTERVENTION

Intervention and Settings

Therapeutic approaches involve psychotherapy (behavioral, cognitive, psychodynamic), sociotherapy, Alcoholics Anonymous (AA) and similar associations, and medications. General Practitioners (GPs) are the key contact figures early on in the intervention for addictive disorders. They see 71% of the general population every year,[6] but their capacity for detecting alcoholism is relatively low. During their education, GPs have limited exposure to a formal drug and addiction curriculum, which limits their effort to initiate treatment, particularly of very difficult problem drinkers.[7] Although minimal intervention programs are encouraged, GPs often refer to specialized agencies both problem drinkers and alcohol-dependent patients. However, about 90% of clients tend not to comply with the referral proposals and thus miss the treatment option.

Detoxification, in Europe, still plays a major part in the initiation of the treatment of alcohol addicts. It is seldom conducted alone but usually integrated by external support (either general psychological or specific psychotherapeutic). The most common procedure is inpatient detoxification at the university clinics or general hospitals, and also in private clinics with a stay no longer than 14 days. GPs rarely intervene directly. Inpatient rehabilitation (for a maximum stay of 3 months) and long-term rehabilitation, performed on an outpatient basis, is provided in most countries, but for a limited number of alcoholics in an advanced state of their "alcoholic career."

Therapeutic Goals

A lack of consensus exists about the goals of therapy which continue to be diverse.[8] Many therapists in the field have as their goal a reduction of problems and an enhancement of health and of personal and social functions, rather than that of abstinence and relapse prevention alone. Suggested goals are to maximize functioning, enhance motivation, restore focus (especially on family well-being), decrease alcohol consumption and achieve relapse prevention.

Counselling and behavioral therapies are more in use in countries where the theoretical therapeutic approach is the reinforcement of the internal more than the external focus of control.[9] In the Mediterranean area, instead, external (social) forces are perceived to be the major determinants of relapse.[10] It follows that, in several European countries where citizens are fully covered by public health plans, sociotherapy is integrated with diverse therapeutic options within programs that are organized at the community level. Attendance at meetings of AA or similar associations (e.g., the Clubs of Treated Alcoholics [CAT])11 becomes a part of a wider long-term rehabilitation program.

AA and CAT groups differ in the definition of addiction, aims and modalities of intervention, and in the relationships existing with the medical system and society at large (Table 2). The CAT treatment model involves large groups including families, community members and different professions.[12] A prolonged follow-up (5 years) is aimed at re-establishing social functions; a result which should also be visible to the entire community.[13] Even though the

TABLE 2. Characteristics of Clubs of Treated Alcoholics (CAT) Groups and Alcoholics Anonymous (AA) Groups

Clubs of Treated Alcoholics	Alcoholics Anonymous
addiction as a family style	addiction as an illness
alcoholics and families	independent family groups
change in lifestyle	12 steps
social functions	no social functions
visibility in the community	anonymity
complex associative structure	no associative structure
± relation with medical system	independent from medical system
± use of drugs (e.g., disulfiram)	no medications
trained therapist	no therapist

question has been raised whether a model developed in the former Yugoslavia could be applied successfully in a different cultural context,[14] in Italy the number of the CAT groups is 4 times greater than AA groups.

PHARMACOLOGICAL INTERVENTION

Pharmacological aids in the treatment of alcoholism could be classified into: (a) drugs treating acute alcohol intoxication, (b) agents treating alcohol withdrawal, and (c) medicaments inhibiting drinking behaviors.

a) Drugs Treating Acute Alcohol Intoxication

Antagonism of acute alcohol intoxication is a lively subject of interest to both clinician and scientist. Of the various substances examined for this purpose, naloxone appears to be the most effective pharmacodynamic antagonist of intoxication. Its use is, however, limited to life threatening situations (coma).[15]

b) Drugs Treating Alcohol Withdrawal

The concomitant presence of withdrawal signs and the fear of complications lead to prescription of medications, even though in proper settings (e.g., in specialized units or also at home under the supervision of a community psychiatric nurse), the need for medications can be markedly reduced.

Drugs enhancing the GABA system, such as the benzodiazepines or the vitamin B derivatives (chlormethiazole[16] and metadoxine[17] which are not present on the American market) are mostly used to prevent seizure episodes.[18] Antiepileptic drugs like carbamazepine[19] and valproic acid[20] (which have been extensively used in Italy since the 1970's) could also serve this purpose. Tiapride[21] is still widely used in Europe. Other drugs like beta-adrenergic blockers,[22] alpha-adrenergic agonists,[23] haloperidol,[24] and calcium-channel blockers[25] are, by contrast, rarely used. Tapered doses of ethanol could also prevent withdrawal signs if given soon after the last alcohol intake. This practice has been progressively replaced by the use of drugs.

The GP rarely initiates detoxification inside his/her practice premises. Even if the GP has advanced screening and treatment experience, accurate studies evaluating outcome of psycho- and pharmacological interventions at GP practices are not available. Reducing subjective discomfort is, indeed, a major behavioral tool to negotiate any future therapeutic intervention, and to increase the probability to refer clients to rehabilitative programs.

c) Drugs Inhibiting Drinking Behaviors

After an alcohol-free interval of 2-3 weeks following detoxification, which is necessary to exclude concomitant psychiatric disturbances, alcohol-dependent patients are ready to enter alcohol rehabilitative programs.

Evaluation of treatment outcome for alcoholics exists at two levels. The informal (in-house program) evaluation, which has been widely used between the 1950's and the 1970's,[26] is not designed to test the effect of medications. It provides information useful to improve the effectiveness of ongoing treatment programs by giving feedback to the staff about the outcome of their efforts. The multisite naturalistic treatment outcome studies,[27-30] however, allow the generalization of results best representing the everyday world of treatment. Formal research (clinical trials) testing the effects of drugs implies double-blind, randomized and placebo-controlled studies. Unfortunately, the most-favoured single-site controlled trial often leads to results having little application to ordinary alcohol treatment programs and common practice. The reasons are the small number of patients, the short duration of study, and the restricted and idealized conditions under which the treatment effect has been investigated. For example, too frequent follow-up visits and tests, far from naturalistic conditions, interfere with motivations of subjects remaining in treatment.

More interesting are the studies involving longer periods (a minimum of 3 months, possibly extended to 6-12 months, with or without the use of the medication). The most powerful conclusions are derived from multisite controlled clinical trials related to long-term rehabilitative programs, which recruit a larger number of subjects. It has been suggested that such trials should not exceed a maximum investigative interval of 12-15 months[31] since life changes assume prominence with time. After two years, treatment accounts for a minimal percentage of the variance in outcome if the life context is not taken into consideration.[32]

For the sake of comparability, using more objective measures and taking into consideration the limits previously discussed, drinking variables are the outcome criteria most used. Examples are quantity and frequency of alcohol consumption, frequency of relapses, the time interval to relapse, the interval from the first drink to full relapse and cumulative abstinence duration.

Two classes of drugs inhibiting drinking behaviors of alcohol dependent subjects exist: (I) enhancing external control, and (II) enhancing internal control through a biological action (Table 3).

Drugs Enhancing External Control

Disulfiram, an aversive agent, acts through the increase of blood acetaldehyde concentrations after ethanol intake producing unpleasant signs (e.g., facial flushing, nausea, vomiting, and tachycardia). A multisite controlled clinical trial[33] proved that the threat of the disulfiram-ethanol reaction was effective in decreasing relapse, and, for the patients who drank, in decreasing the number of drinking days. Disulfiram is thus a psychological (deterrence) treatment as well as a pharmacological (metabolism) one.

Disulfiram, still in use after 45 years, is one of the few demonstrably effective pharmacological tools in alcoholism. When no contraindications apply, it can be integrated to any form of interven-

TABLE 3. Drugs in Use Inhibiting Drinking Behaviors of Alcohol-Dependents

I) Drugs enhancing mechanisms of external control

- Aversive agents: disulfiram

II) Drugs enhancing mechanisms of internal control

- Drugs supposedly stimulating or restoring neurotransmission imbalances in the reward system: tiapride, gamma-hydroxybutyric acid, acamprosate
- Drugs supposedly diminishing the stimulation of the reward system: naltrexone

tion. To maximize external control, it should be given in a "supervised manner" (possibly during group sessions as is given in the Italian CAT system), and the dosage is to be increased when the patient is exposed to high risk situations. Since refusal of intake is considered equivalent to lapse or relapse its use may substitute the need of routine blood ethanol tests, which are sometimes impracticable in certain settings.[34]

Finally, disulfiram could be a very effective tool in the hand of the GP, when the family is included in the therapy for supervision, keeping the patient in treatment, building time to strengthen his motivation, and developing alternative alcohol-free coping techniques.

The other aversive agent: calcium-carbamide is no longer recommended in clinical practice for its adverse effects on patients.[35]

Drugs Enhancing Internal Control

Drugs inhibiting drinking behavior are believed to do so by acting on different neurotransmitters such as serotonin, dopamine, GABA and endogenous opioids. These neurotransmitters have actions that are intimately connected in the meso-cortico-limbic system which is responsible for reinforcing appetitive behaviors.[36]

In this review, studies conducted in alcohol-dependent patients have been grouped into those of: (1) short (12-13 weeks) or (2) long (26-52 weeks) duration.

1. Short-term randomized clinical trials.

Several drugs have been tested in 12-13 weeks trials (Table 4).

The study involving viloxazine had major methodological problems. Drugs which show limited evidence of effect are: tiapride and gamma-hydroxybutyric acid (GHB). Tiapride is an atypical neuroleptic agent which is a selective D_2 receptor antagonist. Its use in preventing relapse has been recently claimed in a study flawed by the lack of standardization of type of psychosocial intervention and of interval of drug intake.[37]

GHB acts as a neurotransmitter or a neuromodulator in concentrations known to be present in animals after ethanol intake. Its neuropharmacological effects include decreasing dopamine functions. This drug (in use only in Italian hospitals) has previously been found effective in the treatment of severe ethanol withdrawal.

TABLE 4. Short Randomized Clinical Trials with Drugs Inhibiting Drinking Behaviors of Alcohol-Dependent Subjects (12-13 weeks follow-up)

Medication	Duration of follow-up (wks)	Number of subjects	Improvement in control	Improvement in treatment	p value	Clinical judgment
Acamprosate	12	85	32	61	< 0.02	positive
Gamma-hydroxy-butyric acid	13	82	19	63	0.001	positive
Naltrexone	12	174	33	68	< 0.01	positive
Tiapride	12	100	30	42	0.001	positive
Viloxazine	12	30	no data	no data	< 0.05	none

Recent studies have also demonstrated a remarkable effect in preventing alcohol relapse in humans. Its possible adverse consequences need to be monitored carefully, because addictive potential, relationship with epilepsy and a brain inborn metabolic defect, and potentiation of the effects of ethanol and benzodiazepines[38,39] have all been reported.

Promising agents are acamprosate and naltrexone. Acamprosate is a synthetic derivative of homotaurinate (calcium bis-acetylhomotaurinate) having a mixed mechanism of action. It interacts with GABA transmission and, has more recently been demonstrated to antagonize the effect of L-glutamate via N-methyl-D-aspartate (NMDA) receptor site. After a first clinical study appearing in 1985, its positive clinical effects have subsequently been replicated in different studies.

Alcohol reinforcing effects are associated with enhanced opioidergic activity in humans, and naloxone in animal models decreased alcohol preference.[40] For this reason, naltrexone, a longer-acting opioid antagonist, has been tested as a part of a comprehensive psychosocial treatment.[41] The effect was most marked in patients who have consumed some alcohol during the study, in those with higher levels of somatic distress, and those more compliant with the treatment program. Another study was able to demonstrate that the effect of naltrexone was carried over, although to a lesser extent, for a period of 6 months after the end of treatment.[42] The use of naltrexone for the treatment of alcohol-dependence has received recent approval by the U.S. Food and Drug Administration (FDA). Naltrexone was approved through a rapid procedure because of its use for more than 20 years in the treatment of heroin addiction and the large database existing on its general safety profile although it is contraindicated in patients with hepatic impairment. Other substances with the same mechanism of action are emerging. Nalmefene is claimed to offer more advantages, because it is not associated to hepatoxicity.[43]

2. Long-term randomized clinical trials.

Trials testing the longer effect (26-52 weeks) of medications have been conducted with several compounds including anxiolytics, dopaminergic drugs and lithium. The drug which proved to have a positive effect has been acamprosate (Table 5).

Buspirone, an interesting non-benzodiazepine anxiolytic having minimal interaction with ethanol, was not associated with significant improvement in outcome in anxious alcohol-dependent subjects. The dopamine agonist, apomorphine, also proved unsuccessful in alcoholism treatment.[44]

The effect of lithium, on the other hand, is controversial. While early studies showed a positive trend, in a more recent, well designed study involving 400 subjects, lithium did not improve outcome for either depressed or nondepressed alcoholic patients.[45] The results are similar to those of disulfiram in that patients in all groups tended to improve with treatment compliance, rather than treatment response being the major predictor. In another study only the patients with lithium concentrations > 0.7 mq/l had a better out-

TABLE 5. Prolonged Randomized Clinical Trials with Drugs Inhibiting Drinking Behaviors of Alcohol-Dependent Subjects (26-52 weeks follow-up)

Medication	Duration of follow-up (wks)	Number of subjects	Improvement in control	Improvement in treatment	p value	Clinical judgment
Buspirone	26	67	55	52	n.s.	negative
Lithium	52	457	28	38	n.s.	none
Apomorphine	26	86	14	10	n.s.	none
Acamprosate	26/52	246	32	48	< 0.01	positive

come.[46] A recent review concluded that the only potential indication of lithium in alcoholism could be the treatment of alcoholism secondary to bipolar affective disorders, but, interestingly, this hypothesis has not been tested so far.[47]

Acamprosate has been tested in a study considering 246 alcohol-dependent subjects in which the drug was given as an adjunct to a community-based alcohol rehabilitation program, and abstinence was approximately 40% higher than in the placebo group. A less significant effect was present 6 months after therapy with the drug was stopped. Positive results on drinking status have been confirmed in 11 trials conducted in different programs throughout Europe where the drug has been used for a period up to one year (around 4,000 patients being involved). Analysis of the data is under way to test if the drug is more effective in different types of alcoholics and/or in combination with other drugs.

Acamprosate has recently received official approval for treating alcoholism in Europe (after a previous approval in France). Studies evaluating the prolonged effect of naltrexone are also underway at present in Europe.

Compared to naltrexone, acamprosate is poorly absorbed and needs frequent daily administration. However, it could be given to heroin addicts and, since it is not hepatotoxic, it is more compatible with other drugs (e.g., disulfiram). A comparison between naltrexone versus acamprosate is shown in Table 6, which gives also the current cost in France. The costs of the drugs in other European

TABLE 6. Comparison Between Promising Drugs Indicated for Alcohol-Dependent Subjects

	Naltrexone	Acamprosate
Approval	U.S.A.	Europe
Dosage	1 tablet/day	6 tablets/day
Pharmacokinetics	bioavailability (40%)	bioavailability (17%)
Interactions	opiates alcohol toxicity	none
Price	$486 × 3 months	$153 × 3 months

countries will clearly depend on market factors and governmental subsidy policies.

The mechanism of action of acamprosate (which supposedly restores the neurotransmission imbalance in the reward system) vs. naltrexone (which suppresses the reinforcing effect of ethanol, and blocks the pleasurable effect or "high" associated with alcohol drinking) will probably limit the effect of naltrexone to more motivated patients.

INTEGRATION OF PHARMACOTHERAPIES WITH PSYCHOSOCIAL TREATMENT

Evidence for the Effectiveness of Psychosocial and Pharmacological Interventions

Psychosocial treatment has been shown to have positive clinical effects.[48] There are systematic data to support that AA effectively helps patients to remain abstinent from alcohol. A recent study reported that individuals who regularly attended AA meetings for one year after either inpatient or outpatient treatment had higher abstinence rates than those individuals who did not.[49] However, in shorter-term follow-up, brief intervention has been shown to be clinically modest, but significant in reducing alcohol intake, and community-based intervention has shown advantages versus conventional hospital management for problem drinkers.[32,50] The CAT programs have also consistently demonstrated fairly good outcomes. Compared to patients who were offered only detoxification, those who had the chance to enter programs remained more abstinent (29.8% versus 8.2% at 12 months).[51] Since the goal of treatment was a change in lifestyle, the results were confirmed on different life functioning variables, and also on clinical outcomes after a 5 year follow-up.[52] The positive outcome was related to the creation of a social support network around the alcoholic patient.

Methods to increase compliance with disulfiram therapy are now available (e.g., intake, under spouse's supervision, or under community reinforcement at each control visit). When naltrexone was given to treat opiate dependence, poor compliance was also observed. When this drug therapy was associated with a psychosocial program for alcoholics, subjects compliant to medication and program did better than non-compliant patients. Also, among compliant patients, the results were significantly better for those taking the substance. Compliance to the program was also increased in patients taking acamprosate according to a naturalistic design[53] with positive effects on drinking outcome. Abstinence and compliance increased at different time intervals in patients receiving acamprosate and psychosocial treatment compared to those under psychosocial treatment only.[54]

Naltrexone has been used in specific populations, but its biological effects are well documented. Acamprosate, on the contrary, has been used in a variety of programs for the treatment of alcoholism in 11 European countries. Treatment modalities varied as treatment outcomes, but still the drug added to the results of the ongoing programs showing an effect overcoming culture-bound aspects. Thus, these studies demonstrate the existence of medicaments able to inhibit drinking behavior and modify the clinical course of alcohol dependence if added to psychosocial intervention.

Interesting additional differentiations started associating a drug to different types of psychosocial intervention among the same clinical population. For example, coping skills and supportive therapy have already been shown to be more effective than no treatment,[55] but, a recent study has shown that the cumulative abstinence rate was highest for patients treated with naltrexone and supportive therapy. For patients who initiated drinking, those who received naltrexone and coping skills therapy were the least likely to relapse into heavy drinking.[42]

CONCLUSION

Types of alcoholics, alcohol programs, and the philosophy underlying treatment approaches vary widely among different countries. However, various psychosocial treatments are effective in improving compliance and in resolving alcohol complications.

At the same time, a combination of different medications with psychosocial therapy is the most rational way to approach alcohol-dependence, since tools to enhance external and internal control are now available. For example, disulfiram could be associated with a drug reducing the reinforcing effect of ethanol and/or a drug stimulating the reward system.

The use of medications is recommended as an adjunct to psychosocial treatment, and it is probable that medications could also be very useful if used by GPs at their practices. This approach is in its initial stage, but is a very promising one since late intervention produces only limited cost-benefit effects.

We are currently witnessing renewed interest in this subject by the pharmaceutical industry. Addictive behaviors (including alcoholism) are the domain of neuroscience for which coherent models and experimental data are available from basic science to clinical medicine. However, helping alcoholics will mean not only persuading the most motivated patients to avoid alcohol totally (in this case drugs other than disulfiram may have little roles to play), but will also mean that all existing tools (psychosocial and biological) will be used to reach the more realistic goals of preventing relapse, reducing the harm caused by alcohol, and ultimately reducing drinking by the alcoholic.

REFERENCES

1. Takala JP, Klingemann H, Hunt G. Afterword: common directions and remaining divergences. In: Cure, care, or control. Alcoholism treatment in sixteen countries. Albany: State University of New York Press, 1992:285-304.

2. The Permanent Observatory on Youth and Alcohol. The institutional and regulatory approach. In: Young people and alcohol in Europe. Rome: Edizioni OTET, 1994:55-92.

3. Roemer MI. National health systems as market interventions. Journal of Public Health Policy 1989; 10:62-77.

4. Porter L, Arif AE, Curran WJ. The law and the treatment of drug and alcohol-dependent persons: a comparative study of existing legislation. Geneva:World Health Organization, 1986.

5. Havard JDJ. Alcohol abuse and legislation in Europe. In: L'Alcologia in Europa. Bologna: Editrice Compositori, 1992:1-12.

6. Anderson P. Management of alcohol problems: the role of the general practitioner. Alcohol Alcohol 1993; 28:263-272.

7. Buchsbaum D. Effectiveness of treatment in general medicine patients with drinking problems. Alcohol Health Res World 1994; 18:140-145.

8. Fuller RK. The assessment of treatment outcome. Alcohol J Alcohol Related Addict 1995; 31:69-77.

9. Rotter J. Generalized expectancies for internal versus external control of reinforcement. Psychol Monogr 1966; 80:1-28.

10. Poldrugo F, Zorzut G. Factors related to alcoholism relapse in an Italian population. Alcohol J Alcohol Related Addict 1991; 27:57-61.

11. Poldrugo F, Urizzi R. The Italian paradox: treatment initiatives and falling alcohol consumption. In: Cure, care, or control. Alcoholism treatment in sixteen countries. Albany, State University of New York Press, 1992:191-204.

12. Patussi V, Tumino E, Poldrugo F. The development of the Alcoholic Treatment Club system in Italy: fifteen years of experience. Contemp Drug Problems 1996; 23:29-42.

13. Bennett L. Treating alcoholics in a Yugoslav fashion. East Eur Q 1985; 18:495-519.

14. Galanter M. Alcoholism programs in the USSR and Yugoslavia: effects of the social context on treatment. In: Currents in Alcoholism. New York: Grune and Stratton, 1981:183-194.

15. Dole VP, Fishman J, Goldfrank L, et al. Arousal of ethanol-intoxicated comatose patients with naloxone. Alcohol Clin Exp Res 1982; 6:275-279.

16. Burrough AK, Morgan MY, Sherlock S. Double-blind controlled clinical trial of bromocriptine, chlordiazepoxide and chlormethiazole for alcohol withdrawal. Alcohol Alcohol 1985; 20:263-271.

17. Bono G, Sinforiani E, Merlo P, et al. Alcoholic abstinence syndromes: short-term treatment with metadoxine. Int J Clin Pharmacol Res 1991; 11:35-40.

18. Poldrugo F, Snead OC. Electroencephalographic and behavioral correlates in rats during repeated ethanol withdrawal syndromes. Psychopharmacology 1984; 83:140-146.

19. Butler D, Messiha FS. Alcohol withdrawal and carbamazepine. Alcohol 1986; 3:113-129.

20. Minuch GI, Rockman GE, German GB, et al. The use of sodium valproate in the treatment of alcoholism. J Addict Dis 1995; 14:67-74.

21. Shaw G, Majumdar S, Waller S, et al. Tiapride in the long-term management of alcoholics of anxious and depressive temperaments. Br J Psychiatry 1987; 150:164-168.

22. Kraus M, Gottlieb L, Horwitz R, et al. Randomized clinical trial of atenolol in patients with alcohol withdrawal. N Engl J Med 1985; 313:905-909.

23. Cushman P. Clonidine and alcohol withdrawal. Adv Alcohol Subst Abuse 1988; 7:17-28.

24. Palestine M, Alatorre E. Control of acute alcoholic withdrawal symptoms: a comparative study of haloperidol and chlordiazepoxide. Curr Ther Res 1976; 20:289-299.

25. Koppi S, Eberardt G, Haller R, et al. Calcium-channel blocking agents in the treatment of acute withdrawal. Caroverine versus meprobamate in a randomized double-blind study. Neuropsychobiology 1987; 17:49-52.

26. Emrick CD. A review of psychologically oriented treatment of alcoholism. II. The relative effectiveness of different treatment approaches and the relative effectiveness of treatment versus no treatment. J Stud Alcohol 1975; 36:88-108.

27. Bromet E, Moos RH, Bliss F, et al. Post-treatment functioning of alcoholic patients: its relation to program participation. J Consult Clin Psychol 1977; 45: 829-842.

28. Polich JM, Armor DJ, Braiker HB. The course of alcoholism: four years after treatment. Santa Monica, Rand Corporation, 1980.

29. Feurlein W, Küfner H. A prospective multicentre study of in-patient treatment for alcoholics: 18- and 48-month follow-up. Eur Arch Psychiatr Neurol Sci 1989; 239:144-157.

30. Miller NS (ed): Treatment of the Addictions: Applications of Outcome Research for Clinical Management. New York: Haworth Press, 1995.

31. The Plinius Major Society. Guidelines on evaluation of treatment of alcohol dependence. Alcohol J Alcohol Related Addict 1994;30 (suppl. 1):1-83.

32. Moos RH, Finney JW, Cronkite RC. Context, coping, and treatment outcome. In: Alcoholism treatment: context, process, and outcome. New York: Oxford University Press, 1990:109-133.

33. Fuller R, Branchey L, Brightwell D, et al. Disulfiram treatment of alcoholism. A Veteran Administration Cooperative Study. JAMA 1986; 256:1449-1455.

34. Allen JP, Litten RZ, Anton R. Measure of alcohol consumption in perspective. In: Measuring alcohol consumption. Psychosocial and biochemical methods. Totowa, Humana Press, 1992:205-226.

35. Vazquez JJ, De Otazu RD, Guillen FJ, et al. Hepatitis induced by drugs used as alcohol aversion therapy. Diagn Histopathology 1983; 6:29-37.

36. Koob G. Drugs of abuse: anatomy, pharmacology and function of reward pathways. Trends Pharmacol Sci 1992; 13:177-184.

37. Shaw GK, Waller S, Majumdar SK, et al. Tiapride in the prevention of relapse in recently detoxified alcoholics. Br J Psychiatry 1994; 165:515-523.

38. Hoes MJ, Vree TB, Guelen PJ. Enhanced plasma concentrations of gamma-hydroxybutyric acid in alcoholics. Br J Addiction 1978; 73:423-424.

39. Mattila MJ, Palva E, Seppala T, et al. Actions and interactions with alcohol of drugs on psychomotor skills: comparison of diazepam and gamma-hydroxybutyric acid. Arch Int Pharmacodyn 1978; 234:236-246.

40. Froehlich JC, Harts J, Lumeng JL, et al. Naloxone attenuates voluntary ethanol intake in rats selectively bred for high ethanol preference. Pharmacol Biochem Behav 1990; 35:385-390.

41. Volpicelli J, Alterman A, Hayashida M, et al. Naltrexone in the treatment of alcohol dependence. Arch Gen Psychiatry 1992; 49:876-880.

42. O'Malley S, Jaffe A, Chang G, et al. Naltrexone and coping skill therapy for alcohol dependence. Arch Gen Psychiatry 1992; 49:881-887.

43. Mason B, Ritvo E, Morgan R, et al. A double-blind placebo-controlled pilot study to evaluate the efficacy and safety of oral nalmefene HCl for alcohol dependence. Alcohol Clin Exp Res 1994; 18:1162-1167.

44. Jensen SB, Christoffersen CB, Noerregaard A. Apomorphine in out-patient treatment of alcohol intoxication and abstinence: a double blind study. Br J Addict 1977; 72:325-330.

45. Dorus W, Ostrow DG, Anton R, et al. Lithium treatment of depressed and nondepressed alcoholics. JAMA 1989; 232:1646-1652.

46. Fawcett J, Clark D, Gibbons R, et al. Evaluation of lithium therapy for alcoholism. J Clin Psychiatry 1984; 45:494-499.

47. Lejoyeux M, Ades J. Evaluation of lithium treatment in alcoholism. Alcohol Alcohol 1993; 28:273-279.

48. Emrick CD, Tonigan JS, Montgomery H, et al. Alcoholics Anonymous: what is currently known? In: Research on Alcoholics Anonymous. New Brunswick, Canada, Alcohol Research Documentation Inc., 1993:41-76.

49. Miller NS, Hoffmann NG: Addictions treatment outcomes. Alcohol Treat Q 1995; 12:41-55.

50. Potamianos G, North WRS, Meade TW, et al. Randomized trial of community-based centre versus conventional hospital management in treatment of alcoholism. Lancet 1986; ii:797-799.

51. Poldrugo F. Evaluation of alcohol treatment programs. In: Proceedings of the international meeting on alcohol and therapy. Gorizia, USL Press, 1993:99-112.

52. Poldrugo F, Chick JD, Moore N, et al. Mortality studies in the long-term evaluation of treatment of alcoholics. Alcohol Alcohol 1993; 28(suppl. 2):151-155.

53. Pelc I, Le Bon O, Verbanck P, et al. Calcium-acetylhomotaurinate for maintaining abstinence in weaned alcoholic patients: a placebo-controlled, double-blind, multicenter study. In: Novel pharmacological interventions for alcoholism. New York, Springer Verlag, 1992:348-352.

54. Poldrugo F, Chabac S, Lehert P. Acamprosate in the long-term treatment of alcoholism: is its use recommended within the psycho-social approach? Alcohol Clin Exp Res 1994; 18:43A.

55. Jones SL, Kanfer R, Lanyon RI. Skills training with alcoholics: a clinical extension. Addict Behav 1982; 7:285-290.

Integration of Research in Pharmacotherapy for Addictive Disease: Where Are We? Where Are We Going?

Walter Ling, MD
Steven Shoptaw, PhD

SUMMARY. Systematic efforts by NIDA and NIAAA to develop new medications for drug and alcohol dependence have resulted in recent FDA approval of LAAM for opiate dependence, naltrexone for alcohol dependence and, more recently, a nasal spray for nicotine dependence. This article reviews the current strategies that guide these development efforts, including further examination of the interactions between potential pharmacotherapeutic agents and the drugs of abuse, the enhancement of pharmacotherapeutic efficacy with non-

---

Walter Ling and Steven Shoptaw are affiliated with the Friends Medical Science Research Center, Inc., Matrix Center, West Los Angeles Veterans Administration Medical Center, and UCLA Department of Psychiatry.

Address correspondence to: Walter Ling, MD, 10350 Santa Monica Boulevard, Suite 340, Los Angeles, CA 90025.

This work is supported in part by NIDA grants R18 DA6082 to Friends Medical Science Research, Inc., and R4408786 to Matrix Center, and by NIDA interagency agreement support to the Medications Development Unit at the West Los Angeles VAMC. The authors wish to thank Sandy Dow for her editorial assistance.

[Haworth co-indexing entry note]: "Integration of Research in Pharmacotherapy for Addictive Disease: Where Are We? Where Are We Going?" Ling, Walter, and Steven Shoptaw. Co-published simultaneously in *Journal of Addictive Diseases* (The Haworth Medical Press, an imprint of The Haworth Press, Inc.) Vol. 16, No. 4, 1997, pp. 83-102; and: *The Integration of Pharmacological and Nonpharmacological Treatments in Drug/Alcohol Addictions* (ed: Norman S. Miller, and Barry Stimmel) The Haworth Medical Press, an imprint of The Haworth Press, Inc., 1997, pp. 83-102. Single or multiple copies of this article are available for a fee from The Haworth Document Delivery Service [1-800-342-9678, 9:00 a.m. - 5:00 p.m. (EST). E-mail address: getinfo@haworth.com].

pharmacological interventions, and the development of more precise and meaningful measures of research outcome. *[Article copies available for a fee from The Haworth Document Delivery Service: 1-800-342-9678. E-mail address: getinfo@haworth.com]*

INTRODUCTION

Since July 1993, the Food and Drug Administration (FDA) has approved three new medications for treating drug dependencies: levo alpha acetyl methadol (LAAM) for opioid dependence, naltrexone (Revia) for alcohol dependence, and, most recently, a nasal spray form of nicotine for nicotine dependence. These recent FDA approvals are the early fruits of coordinated federal support directed toward medication development in this area. In particular, the National Institute on Drug Abuse (NIDA) has set as its top priority the identification, development, and approval of one or more medications for treating cocaine dependence. The National Institute on Alcoholism and Alcohol Abuse (NIAAA), flush from its success in guiding the opioid antagonist naltrexone to market as a treatment for alcohol relapse prevention, is actively evaluating other opioid antagonists and other medications for alcohol dependence treatment. The Medications Development Divisions for both Institutes actively support the identification and evaluation of new medications through the funding of research centers, interagency cooperative research agreements, and individual investigator initiated research. Although NIDA has emphasized the development of a medication for cocaine addiction and NIAAA has focused its attention on continued development of naltrexone and other opioid antagonists, both Institutes continue to emphasize the development and evaluation of novel pharmacotherapies for dependence on opiates, cocaine, amphetamines, alcohol, and nicotine. Other issues pertinent to the development of medications for substance abuse disorders are also being systematically addressed; among them are the studies of interactions between potential pharmacotherapeutic agents and drugs of abuse, enhancement of pharmacotherapeutic efficacy by nonpharmacological interventions, and more meaningful and precise measures of research outcome.

THE MEDICATIONS

It is not our intent to review all of the potential medications being tested or being planned for evaluation. A listing of these medications is provided in Table 1 and the reader will be directed to comprehensive reviews where appropriate. This article aims to provide an overview of the major areas of research emphasis, to highlight some current strategies guiding the development of medications for each of the major drugs of abuse, and to discuss some other important issues still in need of clarification.

Opioid Medications

Medications used to treat opiate addicts can be classified into opioid agonists (methadone, LAAM), partial opioid agonists (buprenorphine, buprenorphine/NX), opioid antagonists (naltrexone), and non-opioid palliative medications (lofexidine, clonidine). Clinically, these medications are targeted for use in treating opiate withdrawal, providing or enhancing opiate maintenance, or preventing relapse.[1] Opioid agonists are restricted to delivery within specialized narcotic treatment clinics for patients with a significant degree of dependence. Partial agonists, mixed agonists/antagonists, and antagonists, less subject to abuse and street diversion, may offer opportunity for use by patients with milder dependence who are being treated in general medical settings. In addition, there is urgent need for a non-narcotic detoxification agent, which can be prescribed by physicians outside the traditional narcotic clinic environment to newly addicted patients or those with mild dependence.

Opioid Agonists

Methadone. Nearly 30 years of research has convincingly established the efficacy and safety of methadone, and particularly methadone maintenance, for treatment for opiate dependence.[2] The best results of mcthadonc maintenance are obtained when treatment is of sufficient duration and with an effective dose, determined by clinical response and, where appropriate, methadone blood level.[3] Methadone maintenance is, for the IV drug user, the most effective

TABLE 1. Medications Evaluated or Under Consideration for Treatment of Opiate, Cocaine, and Alcohol Abuse and Dependence

Drug	Approved Clinical Indication	Opiate Abuse/Dependence[1]	Cocaine Abuse/Dependence[2]	Alcohol Abuse/Dependence[3]
Acetorphan		One of the enkephalinase inhibitors being considered for detoxification; A, RP		
ACPC		Glycine antagonist; D		
Amantadine	Anti-influenza; Anti-Parkinson		Dopamine agonist; RP	
Amoxapin	Antidepressant		Dopamine antagonist, noradrenaline and serotonin reuptake inhibitor; RP	
Baclofen	Anti-spasm		$GABA_B$ agonist; RP	
Benzodiazepines	Anxiolytic	Class of drugs used for symptomatic relief in combination with alpha-2 adrenergic agonists during non-narcotic withdrawal		Class of drugs used to manage acute alcohol withdrawal
Bromocriptine	Anti-Parkinson; hyper-prolactinemia		D2 dopamine receptor agonist; RP, W	D2 dopamine receptor agonist; RP for alcoholics with DRD2 A1 allele
Buprenorphine	Analgesic	Combined mixed opioid agonist/antagonist; M	Combined mixed opioid agonist/antagonist; RP in cocaine dependent opioid addicts	
Buprenorphine/Naloxene		Combined mixed opioid agonist/antagonist with opioid antagonist as diversion protection; M		

A = Adjunct to Maintenance Medication; D = Detoxification; M = Maintenance; RP = Relapse Prevention; W = Withdrawal

Drug	Approved Clinical Indication	Opiate Abuse/Dependence[1]	Cocaine Abuse/Dependence[2]	Alcohol Abuse/Dependence[3]
Buproprion	Antidepressant		Dopamine reuptake inhibitor; RP	
Buspirone	Anxiolytic	5-HT-1_A agonist; A, RP		5-HT-1_A agonist; reduces anxiety in alocholics, but no effect on drinking
Butorphonal	Analgesic	Kappa opioid receptor agonist and mu opioid receptor mixed agonist/antagonist; M		
Butylcholinesterase			Increases metabolism of cocaine; RP	
Calcium acetylhomotaurinate	Alcohol RP (in Europe)			$GABA_A$ agonist, NMDA antagonist; RP
Captopril	Anti-hypertensive	ACE inhibitor; A, RP, W		
Carbidopa/Levodopa	Anti-Parkinson		Precursor of dopamine; inhibits decarboxylation of levodopa peripherally; RP	
Carbamazepine	Anticonvulsant		Reduces polysynaptic responses and blocks posttetanic potentiation; RP	Reduces polysynaptic responses and blocks posttetanic potentiation; W
Citalopram	Antidepressant			Serotonin reuptake inhibitor; RP
Clonidine	Anti-hypertensive	Alpha-2 adrenergic agonist; non-narcotic withdrawal		Alpha-2 adrenergic agonist; W
Cocaine Analogue			Cocaine (coca tea) protocol developed for maintenance	

A = Adjunct to Maintenance Medication; D = Detoxification; M = Maintenance; RP = Relapse Prevention; W = Withdrawal

TABLE 1 (continued)

Drug	Approved Clinical Indication	Opiate Abuse/Dependence[1]	Cocaine Abuse/Dependence[2]	Alcohol Abuse/Dependence[3]
D-Amphetamine	Anorectic		Sympathomimetic amine with CNS stimulant activity; M	
Desipramine	Tricyclic antidepressant		Norephinephrine reuptake blocker; RP, W	
Devazepide		CCK_A antagonist; A, D, RP		
Dextromethorphan	Antitussive	NMDA-receptor antagonist; A, D, RP		
Disulfiram	Antidipsotropic			Inhibits aldehyde dehydrogenase inducing toxic effects; RP
Enadoline		Kappa opioid receptor agonist; A, RP, W		
Ergoloid mesylates	Cognitive enhancer		D1/D2 partial agonist; W	
Fenfluramine	Anorectic		Increases serotonin turnover rates and/or increases glucose utilization; anti-craving medication (RP)	
Fenfluramine/ Phentermine	Anorectic		Fenfluramine (see above); Phentermine is CNS stimulant that elevates blood pressure; multi mechansism for anti-craving (RP)	
Fluoxetine	Antidepressant		Serotonin uptake inhibitor; RP, W	Serotonin uptake inhibitor; RP
Flupenthixol	Antipsychotic		Dopamine antagonist; RP, W	

A = Adjunct to Maintenance Medication; D = Detoxification; M = Maintenance; RP = Relapse Prevention; W = Withdrawal

Drug	Approved Clinical Indication	Opiate Abuse/Dependence[1]	Cocaine Abuse/Dependence[2]	Alcohol Abuse/Dependence[3]
GBR-12909	Tested in Europe as antidepressant anti-Parkinson		Selectively binds to dopamine transporter system; RP	
Gamma-hyrdroxy-butyrate		GABA metabolite; D		
Gepirone	Anxiolytic		5-HT-1_A receptor agonist; RP in primary and methadone maintained	
Ibogaine			NMDA-receptor antagonist with effects on serotonin; may be a relapse prevention medicine. NIDA not actively pursuing ibogaine	
Levo alpha acetyl methadol	Opioid maintenance	Mu opioid receptor agonist; M		
Lamotrigine	Anticonvulsant		Perhaps inhibits voltage dependent sodium channels; RP, W	
Lisuride	Anti-Parkinson; ADHD; hyper-prolactinemia; migraine		Dopamine partial agonist, serotonin antagonist; RP, W	
Lofexidine	Antihypertensive	Alpha-2 adrenergic agonist; A, D, RP, W		Alpha-2 adrenergic agonist; W
Mazindol	Anorectic		CNS stimulant, primarily in limbic system; M, RP, W	
Memantine		NMDA-receptor antagonist being considered for A, D, RP		

A = Adjunct to Maintenance Medication; D = Detoxification; M = Maintenance; RP = Relapse Prevention; W = Withdrawal

TABLE 1 (continued)

Drug	Approved Clinical Indication	Opiate Abuse/Dependence[1]	Cocaine Abuse/Dependence[2]	Alcohol Abuse/Dependence[3]
Methadone	Analgesic; opioid maintenance	Potent mu opioid receptor agonist; M		
Methylphenidate	ADHD		CNS stimulant; M, RP, W for adult ADHD cocaine addicted	
Nalmefene	Reverse opiate overdose			Opioid receptor antagonist; RP
Naltrexone	Reverse opiate overdose; alcohol relapse prevention	Potent mu opioid receptor antagonist; RP	Potent mu opioid receptor antagonist; RP	Potent mu opioid receptor antagonist; RP
Naltrexone (Depot)		Potent mu opioid receptor antagonist in long term delivery format being considered for development for RP		
Nefazodone	Antidepressant		Norepinephrine blocker and 5-HT-2 antagonist; RP, W	
Nimodipine	Anti-stroke	Calcium channel antagonist; A, RP, W		
Ondansetron	Antinausea			5-HT-3 antagonist; RP
Pemoline	ADHD		CNS stimulant; may act through dopaminergic mechanisms; M, RP, W in adult ADHD cocaine addicted	
Pergolide	ADHD		D1/D2 agonist; M, RP, W in adult ADHD cocaine addicted	

A = Adjunct to Maintenance Medication; D = Detoxification; M = Maintenance; RP = Relapse Prevention; W = Withdrawal

Drug	Approved Clinical Indication	Opiate Abuse/Dependence[1]	Cocaine Abuse/Dependence[2]	Alcohol Abuse/Dependence[3]
Phenobarbitol	Anticonvulsant			Non-selective CNS depressant and anticonvulsant; W
Phenytoin	Anticonvulsant		Voltage dependent sodium channel blocker; RP, W	Voltage dependent sodium channel blocker; W
Piracetam			Nootropic (mechanism unknown); RP, W	
Placebo			Inert medication often equivalent to active medication for M, RP, W	Inert medication often equivalent to active medication for M, RP, W
Risperidone	Antipsychotic		D2 antagonist and 5-HT-2 antagonist; RP, W	
SCH-39166; A-66359			D1 dopamine antagonist; RP, W	
Selegeline	Anti-Parkinson		Monoamine oxidase-B inhibitor; RP, W	
Tiapride	Antipsychotic			Selective dopamine D2 receptor antagonist; RP
UH-232; AJ-76; DS-121			Dopamine autoreceptor antagonists; RP, W	
7-Nitroindazole		Nitric oxide synthase inhibitor; D, RP		

[1]Information regarding medications development for opiate abuse and dependence was graciously provided by Barbara Hermann, Ph.D., of NIDA's Medication Development Division.
[2]Information regarding medications development for cocaine abuse and dependence was graciously provided by Dorota Majewska, Ph.D., of NIDA's Medication Development Division and in consultation with Donald Wesson, M.D.
[3]Information regarding medications development for alcohol abuse and dependence was gathered from Litton and Allen's (1995) comprehensive review and a literature review.

intervention for prevention of HIV seroconversion[4] with little fear of disturbance to overall immune function.[5]

While methadone alone is a potent clinical intervention, manipulation of the environment in which it is delivered can have a major influence on its treatment efficacy. Contingent reinforcements have, since the late 1970s, been shown to reinforce abstinence from drug use in methadone maintained patients.[6,7,8,9,10] These contingent reinforcers have ranged from simple opportunities for take home doses to receipt of small amounts of money and tokens.[11,12] Closer examination of the interaction of these treatment enhancement strategies with medication constitutes a significant effort in medication development.

LAAM. Although LAAM (levo alpha acetyl methadol) has been approved by the FDA for treating opioid dependence since July 1993, only a small number of clinics nationwide have instituted its use and its pharmacological and logistic advantages have yet to be realized. Barriers to the implementation of LAAM treatment relate to bureaucratic red tape in rescheduling and in adopting appropriate regulations. General resistance to change and fear of an unfamiliar treatment modality on the part of the clinic personnel have also contributed to the problem. The lesson here may be that future medication development efforts need to include clinical implementation as part of the overall strategy. Several other clinical issues remain, among them the feasibility of take home doses of LAAM and its use in pregnancy, youth, and the medically compromised.

Partial Opioid Agonists

Buprenorphine, Buprenorphine/NX. Considerable data have been accumulated to support the safety and clinical efficacy of buprenorphine. The agonist effect of buprenorphine predominates at low dose and its antagonist effect predominates at high dose, conferring on it a high safety profile with a therapeutic ceiling effect. Higher doses increase its duration of action. Thus far, virtually all the research on buprenorphine for opioid dependence has used the sublingual liquid preparation, a dosage formulation that greatly complicates its clinical delivery. A sublingual combination tablet containing buprenorphine and naloxone (buprenorphine/NX), designed as a take-home medication due to its low risks for diversion and injection abuse, holds promise for use in a general medical setting. A pilot evaluation of the combination tablet has recently been completed.[13] The results, which suggest that it can be delivered with relative ease and is acceptable to patients, are being used to complete planning for a multicenter trial.

As with methadone, patients receiving buprenorphine respond to contingency management procedures. Bickel's group at the University of Vermont has shown that contingent management of the dose significantly reduced illicit drug use in patients maintained on buprenorphine.[14] Buprenorphine also allows for dosing every other day or three times per week.[15] Buprenorphine/NX may be the first long-acting opioid medication that can be safely delivered in a general medication setting. Its relative utility and place in the opioid pharmacotherapeutic armamentarium remains to be established. A sequential model for management of opiate dependent patients is presented in Figure 1.

Non-controlled detoxification agents. The changing scene of heroin addiction and its influence on treatment delivery have stimulated a strong interest in detoxification agents that can be prescribed by physicians in general medical practice. Thus far, clonidine has been the only non-opioid medication available to clinicians that has shown even partial effectiveness in suppressing opioid withdraw-

FIGURE 1. A Sequential Pharmacological Intervention Model for Opiate Dependence

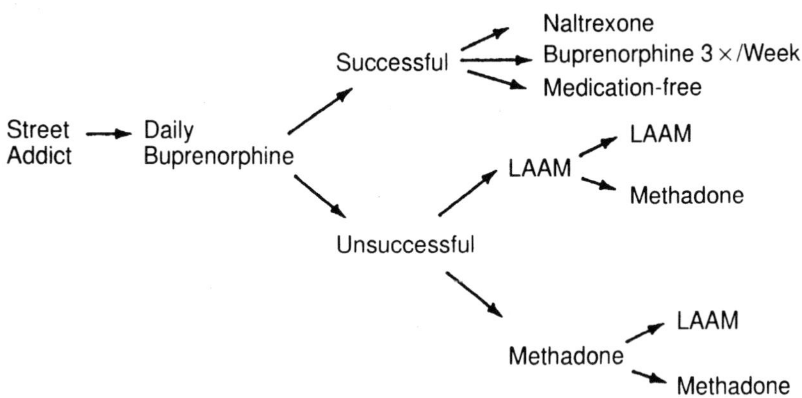

al.[16,17] It has significant side effects, however, especially hypotension and sedation. Lofexidine, chemically related to clonidine, but lacking the hypotensive and sedative side effects, has been in use for detoxification in Great Britain. Although it had been briefly evaluated in the early 1980s, it is not currently available in the US, but there is renewed interest for its full development.

Opioid Antagonists

Naltrexone. Naltrexone, a potent antagonist, can be highly effective in preventing relapse to heroin addiction in certain patients. However, addicts frequently discontinue the medication, leaving themselves vulnerable for resumption of drug use. Behavioral strategies can enhance the treatment results of naltrexone,[18] although long-term outcome is less clear. A depot form of naltrexone could significantly improve clinical compliance.

Ultra-rapid opiate detoxification strategies. Ultra rapid opiate detoxification (UROD) typically involves using general anesthesia or heavy sedation which interferes with the patient's short-term memory (e.g., midazolam). Once anesthetized or sedated, patients are treated with repeated administrations of naloxone, which induces a physiological withdrawal without the patient being aware of the subjective symptoms associated with the withdrawal process. Patients regain consciousness physiologically opiate-free and can begin naltrexone treatment or follow-up care in an abstinence oriented setting.

The place for this detoxification strategy within substance abuse treatment remains to be determined. The process itself requires intensive medical care in an inpatient setting and would thus preclude many addicts who cannot afford to pay. Further, many opiate addicts also use other drugs (estimates range as high as 80%), especially alcohol and cocaine, and may not be suitable for ultra-rapid detoxification for fear of complications. A number of clinicians in this country also question the wisdom of subjecting patients to general anesthesia for what is basically a benign and non-life-threatening medical event. Long-term follow-up data are thus far unavailable. The risk-benefit ratio would warrant reconsideration if it can be shown that long-term follow-up of patients undergoing rapid detoxification demonstrates a lower relapse rate compared to conventional methods of detoxification.

Cocaine Medications

Despite considerable efforts by clinical investigators, the last 15 years of research has yielded no proven efficacious cocaine pharmacotherapies.[19] Recent efforts have focused on medications that initiate and/or facilitate abstinence, treat withdrawal symptoms, and prevent relapse.[20] Many of the drugs evaluated or planned for evaluation share theoretical mechanisms involving the neurobiology of reward. These compounds include direct ligand binders, biogenic amine releasers, biogenic amine uptake blockers, MAO_B inhibitors, dopamine agonists, combined norepinephrine and serotonin uptake blockers, 5-HT-1 agonists, 5-HT uptake blockers, neurotropics, sodium channel blockers, opioid antagonists, opioid mixed agonist/antagonists, calcium channel blockers, and $GABA_B$ agonists.[21]

Unfortunately, medications that have sound theoretical rationale, often supported by pre-clinical data, have not translated into practical clinical utility. The number of medications tried is legend. More recent development efforts have been directed toward identification of novel agents and strategies.

Novel Pharmacotherapies. Novel cocaine treatment agents will likely involve underlying theoretical mechanisms that extend beyond classical reward pathways. Exploratory models that integrate basic science with human laboratory pharmacology might involve identifying new methods for modulating specific subtypes of dopamine and serotonin receptors, identifying new neurotransmitters believed to be involved in cocaine addiction, and identifying biologically based anti-cocaine agents, like enzymes and catalytic antibodies. Such strategies could move beyond traditional pharmacotherapies previously tested into non-traditional (or alternative) pharmacotherapies like nutritional factors, amino acids, neurotransmitter precursors, hormones, antihormones, folk remedies (e.g., kudzu root), Chinese herbal preparations, and hallucinogens (e.g., ibogaine). A number of these agents have been shown in animal studies to reduce cocaine self-administration and have been anecdotally reported to reduce cocaine use in humans. Unfortunately, none has proven safe or efficacious in clinical trials.

Psychostimulants

The urban areas of the West Coast and the Southwest United States have witnessed dramatic increases in methamphetamine abuse since 1990.[22] Because of the subjective effects shared by cocaine and amphetamine/methamphetamine, it has been assumed that medications used to treat cocaine addicts will also be effective for methamphetamine addicts and, likewise, medications ineffective for cocaine will also be ineffective for amphetamines. This may not be the case, however, since the effects of cocaine and amphetamines at the receptor level and beyond may be dissimilar. For example, it appears that inhibition of the 5-HT transporter sites within the serotonin system is inversely related to the re-inforcement effects of amphetamine, and that increased inhibition at these sites results in proportionately decreased reinforcement effect. This does not appear to be the case with cocaine.[23] Also, amphetamine is taken into the nerve terminals and becomes a substrate of dopamine metabolism whereas cocaine remains extracellular.[24] Thus, medications that have not been beneficial for cocaine dependence may yet prove effective for treatment of amphetamine dependence. This realization has prompted re-examination of a number of previously tested agents.

Alcohol

NIAAA continues to investigate naltrexone for treatment of alcoholism and is actively evaluating other opioid antagonists. Nalmefene, an experimental opioid antagonist, appears to provide a more sustained antagonist effect than naltrexone, it does not have a dose dependent association with liver toxicity, and, because of its more effective binding to central opiate receptors, it can be administered in lower doses than naltrexone, thus reducing or eliminating side-effects and increasing treatment retention.[25,26] Acamprosate has demonstrated remarkable efficacy in a number of double-blind, placebo-controlled European trials[27,28] although its mechanism of action remains unspecified.[29] Tiapride, an atypical neuroleptic that works as a selective dopamine D2-receptor antagonist with anxiolytic properties that do not affect vigilance, has also shown considerable promise.[30] The anxiolytic effect of tiapride makes it uniquely useful for acute alcohol withdrawal in place of benzodiazepines, as well as for the prevention of relapse.

Issues remaining regarding the use of naltrexone and other opioid antagonists relate to optimal treatment length and dose, and adjunctive counseling requirements.

Nicotine

Pharmacologic treatment of nicotine dependence has played an important role in smoking cessation over the past two decades. Nicotine polacrilix gum, developed in Sweden, was the first nicotine substitution therapy and has been available since the mid 1970s. The nicotine transdermal patch, shown to be significantly superior to placebo,[31,32,33] has been available for the last five years, and approximates nicotine gum in efficacy. A meta-analysis of several placebo controlled studies of the nicotine patch confirmed its long-term efficacy, compared to placebo, at 6- and 12-month follow-ups.[34] Other forms of nicotine substitution[35] have been studied, including an inhaler which is available in Europe, and a nicotine nasal spray which is now available in Europe and the United States. New nicotine substitution products that are currently under development include a nicotine tablet, a nicotine aerosol ("Eclipse"), and a nicotine toothpick. While these nicotine agonist therapies (gum, patch, inhaler, nasal spray) work on the nicotinic system directly, a number of nicotine antagonist medications, which are currently under investigation, are opposite in action to nicotine substitution therapies. Mecamylamine, which will also be delivered using a transdermal patch in combination with nicotine,[36] is nearing market approval. However, due to its dysphoric effect, mecamylamine suffers from poor treatment compliance. Clonidine and silver salts are two other promising agents that do not involve the nicotinic system directly for their clinical effect.[37,38]

OTHER DEVELOPMENTS

There remain several important issues requiring clarification: the interaction of potential pharmacotherapeutic agents with drugs of abuse, the use of non-pharmacological interventions to enhance pharmacotherapeutic efficacy, and the development and evaluation of more precise and relevant measures of outcome.

Interaction of Drugs of Abuse with Potential Pharmacotherapeutic Agents

Recent interest in developing substitution medications for cocaine and amphetamines has raised concerns about their interactions, especially the increased cardiovascular risks, as well as other side effects that might arise from the use of cocaine or amphetamines during treatment with such medications. Moreover, such medications, methylphenidate for example, may themselves be subject to abuse and diversion, and may "prime" patients to increase rather than decrease drug use. Exploration of novel pharmacotherapeutic strategies, as it proceeds toward clinical evaluation, must also carefully examine such drug-drug interactions in the context of the known pharmacology/chemistry.

Non-Pharmacological Interventions to Enhance Pharmacotherapy Efficacy

Nonpharmacological interventions, such as extent of psychosocial counseling, can affect the outcome of medication efficacy trials. Studies with inadequate psychosocial support may suffer from excessive early patient dropout. Conversely, when medications have small to medium effect sizes, extensive psychosocial intervention may obscure the medication effect. Clinical trial protocols should provide for specification of the extent of psychosocial intervention.

Contingency management, in and of itself, has demonstrated efficacy with opiate[7,8,9,11,12] and cocaine[39,40,41] abusers. As such, it can optimize the results of clinical trials, and knowledge of reinforcers in the context of medication treatments can broaden the application of pharmacotherapies. Designs that allow for assessment of the interaction between the main effects of medication and contingency management will provide more accurate measurement and clearer conclusions regarding the relative efficacy of these treatments.

Relapse prevention, an educational approach that teaches various strategies to prevent drug relapse, has been evaluated as a nonpharmacological strategy for treating a variety of addictive behavior problems. When surveying the literature in total, it seems reasonable to conclude that relapse prevention is a feasible strategy that is generally well accepted by patients seeking treatment. However, studies of relapse prevention have demonstrated less consistent outcomes than those of contingency management. Still, both behavioral strategies have adequate data bases for estimating effect size and represent excellent candidates for integration into pharmacotherapy trials. A number of self-help strategies also enjoy wide acceptance, but their role as adjunctive treatments to medication and their relationship to medication development have yet to be determined.

Methodological Advancements

Measures of patients' responses to medication, either biological or psychosocial, are well standardized, and the Medications Development Divisions of both NIDA and NIAAA have recommended batteries for assessing outcomes. However, the difficult task of aggregating physical measures of drug use, particularly urine toxicology results, continues to daunt researchers. These difficulties include, but are not limited to, such problems as the frequency and sensitivity of toxicology screens, early termination of patients from treatment (or conversely, the continued participation of some patients who respond poorly to treatment), and problems of analyzing a data matrix that contains a large number of missing data points. The Treatment Effectiveness Score (TES), a measure of treatment efficacy that combines retention and urine toxicology results into a single index, is one example of how treatment outcome measures may be simplified and made more clinically meaningful.[42]

REFERENCES

1. Hermann, B. [Clinical Opioid Medications.] Unpublished raw data, 1996.

2. Ball JC, Ross A. The Effectiveness of Methadone Maintenance Treatment. New York: Springer-Verlag, 1991.

3. Martin J, Payte JT, Zweben JE. Methadone maintenance treatment: A primer for physicians. J Psychoactive Drugs. 1991; 23(2):165-176.

4. Moss AR, Vranizan K, Gorter R, Bacchetti P, Watters J, Osmond D. HIV seroconversion in intravenous drug users in San Francisco, 1985-1990. AIDS. 1994; 8:223-231.

5. Kreek MJ. Immune function in heroin addicts and former heroin addicts in treatment: Pre- and post-AIDS epidemic. NIDA Res Monogr. 1990; 96(102): 192-219.

6. Iguchi MY, Stitzer ML, Bigelow GE, Liebson IA. Contingency management in methadone maintenance: Effects of reinforcing and aversive consequences on illicit polydrug use. Drug Alcohol Depend. 1988; 22:1-7.

7. Magura S, Casriel C, Goldsmith D, Strug DL, Lipton DS. Contingency contracting with polydrug-abusing methadone patients. Addict Behav. 1988; 13:113-118.

8. Milby JB, Garrett C, English C, Fritschi O, Clark C. Take home methadone: Contingency effects on drug-seeking and productivity of narcotic addicts. Addictive Behaviors. 1978; 3:215-220.

9. Stitzer MA, Bigelow GE, Liebson IA, Hawthorne JW. Contingent reinforcement for benzodiazepine-free urines: Evaluation of a drug abuse treatment intervention. J Appl Behav Anal. 1982; 15:493-503.

10. Stitzer MA, Iguchi MY, Felch LJ. Contingent take-home incentive: Effects on drug use of methadone maintenance patients. J Consult Clin Psychol. 1992; 60:927-934.

11. Hall SM, Bass A, Hargreaves WA, Loeb P. Contingency management and information feedback in outpatient heroin detoxification. Behav Ther. 1979; 10:443-451.

12. McCaul ME, Stitzer ML, Bigelow GE, Liebson IA. Contingency management interventions: Effects on treatment outcome during methadone detoxification. J Appl Behav Anal. 1984; 17:35-43.

13. Ling W, Huber A, Charuvastra VC, Shoptaw S, Compton P. Buprenorphine/naloxone combination tablet: First clinical experience. Submitted for review 1996.

14. Bickel W. Behavioral treatment enhances outcomes during buprenorphine detoxification. Paper presented at the meeting of the National Institute on Drug Abuse: Workshop on the Behavioral Management of Drug Abuse, Bethesda, MD, Sept. 1995.

15. Amass L, Bickel WK, Higgins ST, Badger GJ. Alternate-day dosing during buprenorphine treatment of opioid dependence. Life Sci. 1994; 54(17):1215-1228.

16. Gold MS, Redmond DE Jr., Kleber HD. Clonidine blocks acute opiate-withdrawal symptoms. Lancet. Sept. 16, 1978, 599-601.

17. Uhde TW, Redmond DE Jr., Kleber HD. Clonidine suppresses the opioid abstinence syndrome without clonidine-withdrawal symptoms: A blind inpatient study. Psychiatry Res.1980; 2(1):37-47.

18. Rawson RA. Contingency management and relapse prevention for primary cocaine users and cocaine-using methadone patients. Paper presented at the meeting of the National Institute on Drug Abuse: Workshop on the Behavioral Management of Drug Abuse, Bethesda, MD. Sept. 1995.

19. Mendelson JH, Mello NK. Management of cocaine abuse and dependence. Drug Ther. 1996; 334(15):965-972.

20. Johnson DN, Vocci F. Medications development at the National Institute of Drug Abuse: Focus on cocaine. In: Tims FM, Leukfeld CG, eds. Cocaine Treatment: Research and Clinical Perspectives. NIDA Res Monogr. 135. NIH Publication No. 93-3639. Washington, DC:US. GPO, 1993:8-56.

21. Majewska D. [Current Cocaine Medications.] Unpublished raw data. 1996.

22. Substance Abuse and Mental Health Services Administration. National Household Survey on Drug Abuse: Population Estimates 1994. 1995.

23. Ritz MC, Kuhar MJ. Relationship between self-administration of amphetamine and monamine receptors in brain: Comparison with cocaine. J Pharmacol Exp Ther. 1990; 248(2):1010-1017.

24. Kuhar MJ. Methamphetamine: Cellular level, mechanism of action. Paper presented at CPDD Satellite Meeting, San Juan, Puerto Rico, June 28, 1996.

25. Fudala PJ, Heishman SJ, Henningfield JE, Johnson RE. Human pharmacology and abuse potential of nalmefene. Clin Pharmacol Ther. 1991; 49: 300-306.

26. Dixon R, Gentile J, Hsu H-B, Hsiao J, Howes J, Garg D, Weidler D. Nalmefene: Safety and kinetics after single and multiple oral doses of a new opioid antagonist. J Clin Pharmacol. 1987; 27:233-239.

27. Lhuintre JP, Moore N, Tran G, Steru L, Langrenon S, Daoust M, Parot P, Ladure P, Libert C, Boismare F, Hillemand B. Acamprosate appears to decrease alcohol intake in weaned alcoholics. Alcohol 1990; 25(6):612-622.

28. Paille FM, Guelfi JD, Perkins AC, Royer RJ, Steru L, Parot P. Double-blind randomized multicentre trial of acamprosate in maintaining abstinence from alcohol. Alcohol. 1995; 30(2):239-247.

29. Littleton J. Acamprosate in alcohol dependence: How does it work? Addiction. 1995; 90:1179-1188.

30. Peters DH, Faulds D. Tiapride. A review of its pharmacology and therepeutic potential in the management of alcohol dependence syndrome. Drugs. 1994; 47(6):1010-1032.

31. Daughton DM, Heatley SA, Prendergast JJ. Effect of transdermal nicotine delivery as an adjunct to low-intervention smoking cessation therapy. Arch Intern Med. 1991; 151:749-752.

32. Fiore MC, Smith SS, Jorenby DE, Baker TB. The effectiveness of the nicotine patch for smoking cessation: A meta-analysis. JAMA. 1994; 274(24):1940-1947.

33. Hughes JR, Glaser M. Transdermal nicotine for smoking cessation. Health Values. 1993; 17:25-31.

34. Sachs DP, Sawe U, Leischow SJ. Effectiveness of a 16-hour transdermal nicotine patch in a medical practice setting, without intensive group counseling. Arch Intern Med. 1993; 153(16):1881-1890.

35. Hjalmarson A, Franzon M, Westin A, Wiklund O. Effect of nicotine nasal spray on smoking cessation. Arch Intern Med. 1994; 154:2567-2572.

36. Rose JE, Behn SM, Westman EC, Levin ED, Stein RM, Ripka GV. Mecamylamine combined with nicotine skin patch facilitates smoking cessation beyond nicotine patch treatment alone. Clin Pharmacol Ther. 1994; 56:86-99.

37. Henningfield JE, Schuh LM, Jarvik ME. Pathophysiology of tobacco dependence. In: Bloom FE, Kipfer DJ, eds. Psychopharmacology: The Fourth Edition, A Generation of Progress. New York: Raven Press, 1995.

38. Gourlay S, Forbes A, Merriner T, Kutin J, McNeil J. A placebo-controlled study of three clonidine doses for smoking cessation. 1994; 55:64-69.

39. Higgins ST, Budney AJ, Bickel WK, Foerg FE, Donhan R, Badjer GJ. Incentives improve outcome in outpatient behavioral treatment of cocaine dependence. Arch Gen Psychiatry. 1994; 51(7):568-576.

40. Higgins ST, Delaney DD, Budney AJ, Bickel WK, Hughes JR, Foerg F, Fenwick JW. A behavioral approach to achieving initial cocaine abstinence. Am J Psychiatry. 1991; 148:1218-1224.

41. Silverman K, Higgins ST, Brooner RK, Montoya ID, Cohen EJ, Schuster CR, Preston KL. Sustained cocaine abstinence in methadone maintained patients through voucher based reinforcement therapy. Arch Gen Psychiatry. 1996; 53:409-415.

42. Ling W, Shoptaw S, Wesson D, Rawson RA, Compton M, Klett CJ. Treatment Effectiveness Score as an outcome measure in clinical trials. NIDA Res Monogr. In press.

SELECTIVE GUIDE TO CURRENT REFERENCE SOURCES ON TOPICS DISCUSSED IN THIS ISSUE

Integration of Pharmacological and Nonpharmacological Treatments in Drug/Alcohol Addictions

Lynn Kasner Morgan, MLS

Each issue of *Journal of Addictive Diseases* features a section offering suggestions on where to look for further information on included topics. The intent is to guide readers to selective substantive sources of current information.

Some published reference works utilize designated terminology

Lynn Kasner Morgan is Assistant Professor of Medical Education, Assistant Dean for Information Resources and Systems, and Director of the Gustave L. and Janet W. Levy Library of the Mount Sinai Medical Center, Inc., One Gustave L. Levy Place, New York, NY 10029-6574.

[Haworth co-indexing entry note]: "Selective Guide to Current Reference Sources on Topics Discussed in This Issue." Morgan, Lynn Kasner. Co-published simultaneously in *Journal of Addictive Diseases* (The Haworth Medical Press, an imprint of The Haworth Press, Inc.) Vol. 16, No. 4, 1997, pp. 103-115; and: *The Integration of Pharmacological and Nonpharmacological Treatments in Drug/ Alcohol Addictions* (ed: Norman S. Miller, and Barry Stimmel) The Haworth Medical Press, an imprint of The Haworth Press, Inc., 1997, pp. 103-115. Single or multiple copies of this article are available for a fee from The Haworth Document Delivery Service [1-800-342-9678, 9:00 a.m. - 5:00 p.m. (EST). E-mail address: getinfo@haworth.com].

(controlled vocabularies) which must be used to find material on topics of interest. For these, a sample of available search terms has been indicated to assist the reader in accessing appropriate sources for his/her purposes. Other reference tools use keywords or free text terms from the title of the document, the abstract, and the name of any responsible agency or conference. In searching using keywords, be sure to look under all possible synonyms to retrieve the concept in question.

An asterisk (*) appearing before a published source indicates that all or part of that source is in machine-readable form and can be accessed through an online database search. Database searching is recommended for retrieving sources of information that coordinate multiple variables, concepts, or subject areas. Most health sciences libraries offer database services which can include mediated online searching, access to locally mounted datafiles, front-end software packages, and CD-ROM technology. Searching can also be done from one's office or home with subscriptions to database service vendors and microcomputers equipped with modems.

Interactive electronic communications systems, such as electronic mail, discussion groups, bulletin boards, and receiving and transferring files are available through the Internet, which offers timely and global information resources in all disciplines, including the health sciences. Some groups which might be of interest are: ALCOHOL (ALCOHOL@LMUACAD), DRUG ABUSE (DRUGABUS@UMAB), 12STEP@TRWRB.DSD.COM and ADDICTION MEDICINE (MAJORDOMO@AVOCADO.PC.HELSINKI.FI). The National Clearinghouse for Alcohol and Drug Information Center for Substance Abuse Prevention maintains PREVLINE, a bulletin board for alcohol and drug information. Information from PREVLINE is available through the Internet at www.health.org and a recent search included such things as results of the 1995 National Household Survey on Drug Abuse. There are also many sites with World Wide Web pages which can be reached by individuals with a Web browser such as Mosaic or Netscape. Netscape "net search" allows searching with many different web search engines. Suggested starting points are http://www.yahoo.com/health, Web Crawler searching tool http://webcrawler.com or World Wide Web Worm http://wwwmcb.cs.colorado.edu/home/mcbryan/wwww.html. Other sites to try include:

Web of Addictions at http://www.well.com/user/woa; American Psychological Association Division of Pharmacology and Substance Abuse at http://charlotte.med.nyu.edu/woodr/div28.html; and Online AA resources at http://www.recovery.org. The amount of information available on the Internet increases daily and attention should be given to the author/provider of the information, which ranges from highly respected institutions to individuals with a home computer and a desire to "publish."

Readers are encouraged to consult their librarians for further assistance before undertaking research on a topic.

Suggestions regarding the content and organization of this section are welcome and should be sent to the author.

1. INDEXING AND ABSTRACTING SOURCES

Place of publication, publisher, start date, frequency of publication, and brief descriptions are noted.

**Biological Abstracts* (1926-) and *Biological Abstracts/RRM* (v.18, 1980-). Philadelphia, BioSciences Information Service, semimonthly. Reports on worldwide research in the life sciences.

See: Concept headings for abstracts, such as behavioral biology, pharmacology, psychiatry, public health, and toxicology sections.

See: Keyword-in-context subject index.

**Chemical Abstracts*. Columbus, Ohio, American Chemical Society, 1907- , weekly. A key to the world's literature of chemistry and chemical engineering, including serial publications, proceedings and edited collections, technical reports, dissertations, new book and audiovisual materials announcements, and patent documents.

See: *Index Guide* for cross-referencing and indexing policies.

See: *General Subject Index* terms, such as drug dependence, drug-drug interactions, drug tolerance.

See: Keyword subject indexes.

**Dissertation Abstracts International. Section A. The Humanities and Social Sciences and Section B. The Sciences and Engineering.* Ann Arbor, Mich., University Microfilms, v.30, 1969/70- , monthly. Includes author-prepared abstracts of doctoral dissertations from 500 participating institutions throughout North America and the world. A separate section contains European dissertations.

See: Keyword subject index.

**Excerpta Medica.* Amsterdam, The Netherlands, Excerpta Medica Foundation, 1947- , 42 subject sections.

A major abstracting service covering more than 4,300 biomedical journals. The abstracts, including English summaries for non-English-language articles, appear in one or more of the published subject sections, excluding Section 38, *Adverse Reactions Titles,* which is an index only. Each of the sections has a comprehensive subject index. Since 1978 all the *Excerpta Medica* sections have been available for computer searching in the integrated online file, EMBASE. Particularly relevant to the topics in this issue are Section 40, *Drug Dependence, Alcohol Abuse and Alcoholism*; and the sections that have addiction, alcoholism, or drug subdivisions: Section 30, *Clinical and Experimental Pharmacology*; Section 32, *Psychiatry*; and Section 17, *Public Health, Social Medicine and Epidemiology.*

**Hospital and Health Administration Index.* Chicago, American Hospital Association, v.51, 1995- three issues per year, with annual cumulations. Published as the primary guide to literature on the organization and administration of hospitals and other healthcare providers, the financing and delivery of healthcare, the development and implementation of health policy and reform, and health planning and research.

See: *MeSH* terms, such as alcoholism; comorbidity; heroin dependence; methadone; psychotropic drugs; substance abuse; substance abuse detection; substance abuse treatment centers; substance dependence; substance withdrawal syndrome.

**Index Medicus* (includes *Bibliography of Medical Reviews*). Bethesda, Md., National Library of Medicine, 1960- , monthly, with annual cumulations. Published as author and subject indexes to more than 3,000 journals in the biomedical sciences. Subject headings are based on the controlled vocabulary or thesaurus, *Medical Subject Headings (MeSH).*

Since 1966 it has been produced from the MEDLARS database, which provides more comprehensive retrieval, including keyword access and English-language abstracts, than its printed counterparts: *Index Medicus*, *International Nursing Index*, and *Index to Dental Literature*.

See: *MeSH* terms, such as alcohol drinking; alcoholism; alcoholic intoxication; comorbidity; heroin dependence; metabolic detoxification; drug; methadone; substance abuse; substance abuse treatment centers; substance dependence; substance withdrawal syndrome.

Index to Scientific Reviews. Philadelphia, Institute for Scientific Information, 1974- , semiannual.

See: Permuterm keyword subject index.

See: Citation index.

**International Pharmaceutical Abstracts*. Washington, D.C., American Society of Hospital Pharmacists, 1964- , semimonthly. A key to the world's literature of pharmacy.

See: IPA subject terms, such as alcoholism; controlled substances; dependence; drug abuse; drug withdrawal; methadone; opiates; pharmacotherapy.

See: Subject sections legislation, laws and regulations; sociology, economics and ethics; toxicology.

**Psychological Abstracts*. Washington, D.C., American Psychological Association, 1927- , monthly. A compilation of nonevaluative summaries of the world's literature in psychology and related disciplines.

See: Index terms, such as addiction; alcohol abuse; alcoholism; alcohol rehabilitation; comorbidity; drug abuse; drug addiction; drug dependency; drug rehabilitation; drug therapy; drug usage; drug usage screening; drug withdrawal; methadone; opiates; psychopharmacology; social issues; treatment outcomes.

**Public Affairs Information Service Bulletin*. New York, Public Affairs Information Service, v.55, 1969- , semimonthly. An index to library material in the field of public affairs and public policy published throughout the world.

See: PAIS subject headings, such as alcoholism; drug abuse; drug addicts; drugs.

**Science Citation Index*. Philadelphia, Institute for Scientific Information, 1961- , bimonthly.

See: Permuterm keyword subject index.

See: Citation index.

**Social Planning/Policy & Development Abstracts*. San Diego, Calif., Sociological Abstracts, Inc., v.6, 1984- , semi-annual.

See: Thesaurus and descriptors listed under *Sociological Abstracts.*

**Social Work Abstracts*. New York, National Association of Social Workers, v.13, 1977- , quarterly.

See: Subject index.

**Sociological Abstracts*. San Diego, Calif., Sociological Abstracts, Inc., 1952- , 6 times per year. A collection of nonevaluative abstracts which reflect the world's serial literature in sociology and related disciplines.

See: *Thesaurus of Sociological Indexing Terms.*

See: Descriptors such as addict/addicts/addicted/addictive/addiction; alcohol abuse; alcoholism; detoxification; drinking behavior; drug abuse; drug addiction; drug use; methadone maintenance; opiates; substance abuse.

2. CURRENT AWARENESS PUBLICATIONS

**Current Contents: Clinical Medicine*. Philadelphia, Institute for Scientific Information, v.15, 1987- , weekly.

See: Keyword index.

**Current Contents: Life Sciences*. Philadelphia, Institute for Scientific Information, v.10, 1967- , weekly.

See: Keyword index.

**Current Contents: Social & Behavioral Sciences*. Philadelphia, Institute for Scientific Information, v.6, 1974- , weekly.

See: Keyword index.

3. BOOKS

**Medical and Health Care Books and Serials in Print: An Index to Literature in the Health Sciences*. New York, R. R. Bowker Co., annual.

See: Library of Congress subject headings, such as alcoholism; drug abuse; drugs; hospitals-outpatient services; methadone maintenance; narcotic habit; pharmacology; substance abuse.

**National Library of Medicine Current Catalog*. Bethesda, Md., National Library of Medicine, 1966- , quarterly, with annual cumulations.

See: MeSH terms as noted in Section 1 under *Index Medicus.*

Bellenir, Karen. *Substance Abuse Sourcebook.* Detroit, Omnigraphics, 1996.

O'Brien, Robert [and others]. *The Encyclopedia of Drug Abuse.* 2nd ed. New York, Facts on File, c1992.

Stimmel, Barry [and others]. *The Facts About Drug Use: Coping with Drug Use in Your Family, at Work, in Your Community.* Mount Vernon, N.Y., Consumers' Union, c1991.

Substance Abuse: The Nation's Number One Health Problem, Key Indicators for Policy. Princeton, N.J., Robert Wood Johnson Foundation, 1993.

Kinney, Jean. *Clinical Manual of Substance Abuse.* St. Louis, Mosby, 1996.

World Health Organization Catalogue: New Books. Geneva, World Health Organization, semiannual (supplements *World Health Organization Publications* and includes periodicals).

See Also: http://www.who.org

4. U.S. GOVERNMENT PUBLICATIONS

Alcohol and Other Drug Thesaurus: A Guide to Concepts and Terminology in Substance Abuse and Addiction (AOD Thesaurus). Rockville, Md., National Institute on Alcohol Abuse and Alcoholism, 1993.

See: Title keyword index.

**Monthly Catalog of United States Government Publications.* Washington, D.C., U.S. Government Printing Office, 1895- , monthly.

See: Keyword index.

See Also: http://www.access.gpo.gov

5. ONLINE BIBLIOGRAPHIC DATABASES

Only those databases which have no print counterparts are included in this section. Print sources which have online database equivalents are noted throughout this guide by the asterisk (*) which appears before the title. If you do not have direct access to these databases, consult your librarian for assistance.

ALCOHOL AND ALCOHOL PROBLEMS SCIENCE DATABASE: ETOH (National Institute on Alcohol Abuse and Alcoholism, Rockville, Md.).

Use: Keywords.

ALCOHOL INFORMATION FOR CLINICIANS AND EDUCATORS (Project Cork Institute, Dartmouth Medical School, Hanover, N.H.)

Use: Keywords.

See Also: http://www.dartmouth.edu/dms/cork

AMERICAN STATISTICS INDEX (ASI) (Congressional Information Services, Inc., Washington, D.C.).

Use: Keywords.

DRUG INFORMATION FULLTEXT (American Society of Hospital Pharmacists, Bethesda, Md.).

Use: Keywords.

DRUGINFO AND ALCOHOL USE AND ABUSE (Hazelden Foundation, Center City, Minn., and Drug Information Service Center, College of Pharmacy, University of Minnesota, Minneapolis, Minn.).

Use: Keywords.

See Also: http://www.hazelden.org

LEXIS (LEXIS-NEXIS, Dayton, Ohio).

Use: Guide library.

MAGAZINE INDEX (Information Access Co., Foster City, Calif.).

Use: Keywords.

MENTAL HEALTH ABSTRACTS (MHA) (IFI/Plenum Data Co., Wilmington, NC).

Use: Keywords.

NATIONAL NEWSPAPER INDEX (Information Access Co., Foster City, Calif.).

Use: Keywords.

NTIS (Bibliographic Data Base, U.S. National Technical Information Service, Springfield, Va.).

Use: Keywords.

PSYCINFO (American Psychological Association, Washington, D.C.).

Use: Keywords.

WESTLAW (West Publishing Co., Eagan, Minn.)

Use: Keywords.

6. HANDBOOKS, DIRECTORIES, GRANT SOURCES, ETC.

Annual Register of Grant Support. Wilmette, Ill., National Register Pub. Co., annual.

See: Internal medicine; medicine; pharmacology, psychiatry, psychology, mental health sections.

See: Subject index.

**Biomedical Index to PHS-Supported Research.* Bethesda, Md., National Institutes of Health, Division of Research Grants, annual.

See: Subject index.

**Database Directory.* White Plains, N.Y., Knowledge Industry Publications in cooperation with the American Society for Information Science, annual.

See: Subject index.

Directory of Research Grants. Phoenix, Ariz., Oryx Press, annual.

See: Subject index terms, such as alcohol/alcoholism, education, drugs/drug abuse, health promotion.

**Encyclopedia of Associations.* Detroit, Gale Research Co., annual (occasional supplements between editions).

See: Subject index.

**Foundation Directory.* New York, The Foundation Center, biennial (updated between editions by *Foundation Directory Supplement*).

See: Index of foundations.

See: Index of foundations by state and city.

See: Index of donors, trustees, and administrators.

See: Index of fields of interest.

See Also: http://www.fdncenter.org

**Health Hotlines: Toll-Free Numbers from DIRLINE*. Bethesda, Md., National Library of Medicine, biennial.

Information Industry Directory. Detroit, Gale Research Co., annual.

Nolan, Kathleen Lopez. *Gale Directory of Databases*. Detroit, Gale Research, Inc., 1995.

Roper, Fred W. and Jo Anne Boorkman. *Introduction to Reference Sources in the Health Sciences*. 3rd ed. Chicago, Medical Library Association, c1994.

The SALIS Directory: Substance Abuse Librarians and Information Specialists. 2nd ed. Berkeley, Calif., Alcohol Research Group, Medical Research Institute of San Francisco and University of California, Berkeley, 1991.

Statistics Sources. 19th ed. Detroit, Gale Research Inc., 1996.

7. JOURNAL LISTINGS

**The Serials Directory. An International Reference Book*. Birmingham, Ebsco Publishing, annual (supplemented by quarterly updates).

**Ulrich's International Periodicals Directory, Now Including Irregular Serials & Annuals*. New York, R. R. Bowker Co., annual (updated between editions by *Ulrich's Quarterly*).

See: Subject categories, such as drug abuse and alcoholism, medical sciences, pharmacy and pharmacology, psychology, public health and safety.

8. AUDIOVISUAL PROGRAMS

The Directory of Medical Video Programs. Hawthorne, N.J., Ridge Publishing Co., 1990.

**National Library of Medicine Audiovisuals Catalog*. Bethesda, Md., National Library of Medicine, 1977-1993, quarterly, with annual cumulations.

See: *MeSH* terms as noted in Section 1 under *Index Medicus.*

Patient Education Sourcebook. 2v. Saint Louis, Mo., Health Sciences Communications Association, c1985-90.

See: *MeSH* terms as noted in Section 1 under *Index Medicus.*

9. GUIDES TO UPCOMING MEETINGS

Scientific Meetings. San Diego, Calif., Scientific Meetings Publications, quarterly.

See: Subject indexes.

See: Association listing.

World Meetings: Medicine. New York, Macmillan Pub. Co., quarterly.

See: Keyword index.

See: Sponsor directory and index.

World Meetings: Outside United States and Canada. New York, Macmillan Pub. Co., quarterly.

See: Keyword index.

See: Sponsor directory and index.

World Meetings: United States and Canada. New York, Macmillan Pub. Co., quarterly.

See: Keyword index.

See: Sponsor directory and index.

10. PROCEEDINGS OF MEETINGS

**Directory of Published Proceedings. Series SEMT. Science/Engineering/Medicine/Technology.* Harrison, N.Y., InterDok Corp., v.3, 1967- , monthly, except July-August, with annual cumulations.

**Index to Scientific and Technical Proceedings*. Philadelphia, Institute for Scientific Information, 1978- , monthly with semiannual cumulations.

11. SPECIALIZED RESEARCH CENTERS

Medical Research Centres. Harlow, Essex, Longman, biennial.

International Research Centers Directory. Detroit, Gale Research Co., annual.

Research Centers Directory. Detroit, Gale Research Co., annual (updated by *New Research Centers*).

12. SPECIAL LIBRARY COLLECTIONS

Directory of Special Libraries and Information Centers. Detroit, Gale Research Co., annual (updated by *New Special Libraries*).

Index

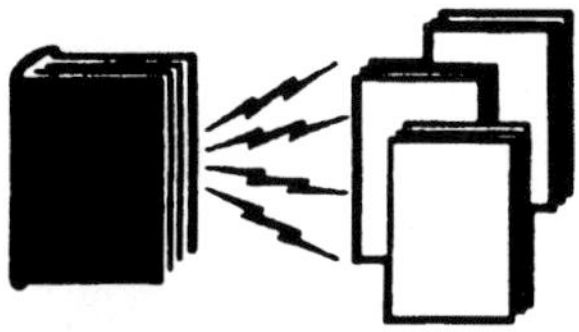

Haworth DOCUMENT DELIVERY SERVICE

This valuable service provides a single-article order form for any article from a Haworth journal.

- *Time Saving:* No running around from library to library to find a specific article.
- *Cost Effective:* All costs are kept down to a minimum.
- *Fast Delivery:* Choose from several options, including same-day FAX.
- *No Copyright Hassles:* You will be supplied by the original publisher.
- *Easy Payment:* Choose from several easy payment methods.

Open Accounts Welcome for . . .
- Library Interlibrary Loan Departments
- Library Network/Consortia Wishing to Provide Single-Article Services
- Indexing/Abstracting Services with Single Article Provision Services
- Document Provision Brokers and Freelance Information Service Providers

MAIL or *FAX* THIS ENTIRE ORDER FORM TO:

Haworth Document Delivery Service
The Haworth Press, Inc.
10 Alice Street
Binghamton, NY 13904-1580

or FAX: 1-800-895-0582
or CALL: 1-800-342-9678
9am-5pm EST

PLEASE SEND ME PHOTOCOPIES OF THE FOLLOWING SINGLE ARTICLES:

1) Journal Title: ______________________________
Vol/Issue/Year: ______________ Starting & Ending Pages: ____________
Article Title: ______________________________
____

2) Journal Title: ______________________________
Vol/Issue/Year: ______________ Starting & Ending Pages: ____________
Article Title: ______________________________
____

3) Journal Title: ______________________________
Vol/Issue/Year: ______________ Starting & Ending Pages: ____________
Article Title: ______________________________
____

4) Journal Title: ______________________________
Vol/Issue/Year: ______________ Starting & Ending Pages: ____________
Article Title: ______________________________
____

(See other side for Costs and Payment Information)

COSTS: Please figure your cost to order quality copies of an article.

1. Set-up charge per article: $8.00
   ($8.00 × number of separate articles) __________
2. Photocopying charge for each article:
   1-10 pages: $1.00 __________
   11-19 pages: $3.00 __________
   20-29 pages: $5.00 __________
   30+ pages: $2.00/10 pages __________
3. Flexicover (optional): $2.00/article __________
4. Postage & Handling: US: $1.00 for the first article/
   $.50 each additional article __________
   Federal Express: $25.00 __________
   Outside US: $2.00 for first article/
   $.50 each additional article __________
5. Same-day FAX service: $.35 per page __________

GRAND TOTAL: __________

METHOD OF PAYMENT: (please check one)

❑ Check enclosed ❑ Please ship and bill. PO # __________
(sorry we can ship and bill to bookstores only! All others must pre-pay)

❑ Charge to my credit card: ❑ Visa; ❑ MasterCard; ❑ Discover; ❑ American Express;

Account Number: __________ Expiration date: __________

Signature: ✗ __________

Name: __________ Institution: __________

Address: __________

____

City: __________ State: __________ Zip: __________

Phone Number: __________ FAX Number: __________

MAIL or *FAX* THIS ENTIRE ORDER FORM TO:

Haworth Document Delivery Service
The Haworth Press, Inc.
10 Alice Street
Binghamton, NY 13904-1580

or FAX: 1-800-895-0582
or CALL: 1-800-342-9678
9am-5pm EST)